STUDY GUIDE AND SELF-EXAMINATION REVIEW FOR

CORE TEXT OF NEUROANATOMY

THIRD EDITION

STUDY GUIDE AND SELF-EXAMINATION REVIEW FOR

CORE TEXT OF NEUROANATOMY

THIRD EDITION

MALCOLM B. CARPENTER, A.B., M.D.

Professor of Anatomy
F. Edward Hébert School of Medicine
Uniformed Services University of the Health Sciences
Bethesda, Maryland

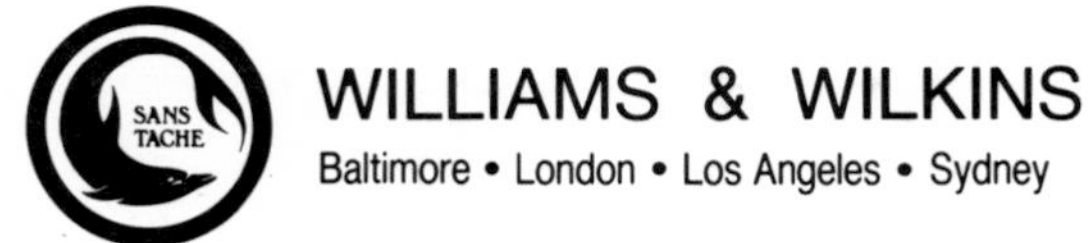

WILLIAMS & WILKINS
Baltimore • London • Los Angeles • Sydney

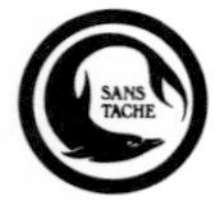

Editor: John N. Gardner
Associate Editor: Victoria M. Vaughn
Copy Editor: William Vinck
Design: JoAnne Janowiak
Illustration Planning: Wayne J. Hubbel
Production: Raymond E. Reter

Printed in the United States of America

Library of Congress Cataloging in Publication Data
Carpenter, Malcolm B.

Study guide and self-examination review for Core text of neuroanatomy, third edition.

1. Neuroanatomy—Examinations, questions, etc. I. Carpenter, Malcolm B. Core text of neuroanatomy. 3rd ed. II. Title. [DNLM: 1. Neuroanatomy—examination questions. WL 101 C296c Suppl.]
QM451.C374 1985 611′.8′076 85-6263
ISBN 0-683-01456-0

Composed and printed at the
Waverly Press, Inc.

85 86 87 88 89
10 9 8 7 6 5 4 3 2 1

Preface

This *Study Guide and Self-examination Review* is designed as a companion to the third edition of the *Core Text of Neuroanatomy.* The purpose of the study guide is to permit self-examination and self-evaluation of the effectiveness of reading, attending lectures, and participating in laboratory exercises. Questions are grouped in 12 sections which in general correspond to the chapter sequence in the *Core Text of Neuroanatomy.* Some sections cover material in more than one chapter of the text and some questions are based on material appearing in several chapters. All questions are prepared in the format used by national testing services. Four types of questions are presented: (1) one best response, (2) "matching," (3) multiple true-false comparison, and (4) multiple true-false. The order in which questions appear in the various sections is random and does not correspond to the organization of material in any chapter. Simple drawings and some photomicrographs have been used to increase the value of certain questions. If questions are well constructed, they can provide a real learning experience and sometimes a much better understanding of the material. Attempts have been made to avoid "trick" questions, to avoid overly complex, wordy questions, and to avoid answers that may be ambiguous or unclear. Questions which form the basis of this study guide have been developed over a long period of teaching experience in collaboration with teaching associates. No claim is made that the questions are the work of a single author. Credit by association must be given to many colleagues, chief among these is Professor Charles R. Noback of the College of Physicians and Surgeons, Columbia University. Credit also is due my teaching associates at the Uniformed Services University, namely Professors Rosemary Borke, Rita P. C. Liu, and Donald B. Newman. Professor Robert R. Batton III of Marshall University assembled and categorized many questions used over the years and special thanks is due for this effort. All questions have been carefully edited, revised, and selected by the author on the basis of their value in helping the student to understand the most complex system of the body. Answers and explanations of the questions are provided in a separate section. If the answer is straightforward and comes directly from the text, no explanation is provided, but a page citation may be given. If the question is more complex, involves problem solving, or the synthesis of material from several sources, the answer and a brief explanation are provided along with page citations.

The author acknowledges with thanks the photographic material generously provided by Professor Duane E. Haines of West Virginia University. For the use of the original plates from H. A. Riley's *Atlas of the Basal Ganglia, Brain Stem and Spinal Cord*, the author is indebted to the late Professor Fred A. Mettler and Williams & Wilkins. Martin Nau of the Uniformed Services University provided invaluable art work and Antonio B. Pereira prepared the photographic material. The manuscript was carefully prepared and typed by Mrs. Doris Lineweaver of Pennsylvania State University at Hershey. It is hoped that this study guide will prove useful for first-year medical students and to those more advanced in their training who are preparing for other examinations.

Malcolm B. Carpenter, M.D.

Contents

Preface v

Section 1 MENINGES, CEREBROSPINAL FLUID, AND GROSS BRAIN 1
Answers 15

Section 2 SPINAL CORD 17
Answers 36

Section 3 MEDULLA 39
Answers 51

Section 4 PONS 53
Answers 67

Section 5 MESENCEPHALON 71
Answers 84

Section 6 CEREBELLUM 87
Answers 100

Section 7 DIENCEPHALON AND THALAMUS 103
Answers 122

Section 8 HYPOTHALAMUS 125
Answers 133

Section 9 CORPUS STRIATUM AND RELATED NUCLEI 135
Answers 148

Section 10 OLFACTORY PATHWAYS, HIPPOCAMPAL FORMATION, AND AMYGDALA 151
Answers 159

Section 11 CEREBRAL CORTEX 161
Answers 171

Section 12 BLOOD SUPPLY OF THE CENTRAL NERVOUS SYSTEM 173
Answers 180

1

Meninges, Cerebrospinal Fluid, and Gross Brain

Questions

Select the one best answer

1.1. Broca's speech area is:
(A) the inferior frontal gyrus
(B) present on both banks of the lateral sulcus
(C) represented bilaterally
(D) the pars opercularis and pars triangularis of the dominant hemisphere
(E) found in the nondominant hemisphere

1.2. The posterior limb of the internal capsule lies between:
(A) the caudate nucleus and the putamen
(B) the thalamus and the putamen
(C) the hypothalamus and the thalamus
(D) the thalamus and the globus pallidus
(E) the thalamus and the crus cerebri

1.3. The compact bundle of fibers originating in part from the hippocampal formation and arching over the thalamus is the:
(A) corpus callosum
(B) anterior commissure
(C) fornix
(D) posterior commissure
(E) habenula

1.4. Hydrocephalus due to aqueductal obstruction could be relieved best by:
(A) removal of the choroid plexus in the lateral ventricles
(B) a shunt from the lateral ventricle to either the cisterna magna or the right atrium of the heart
(C) drainage from the cisterna magna
(D) perforation of the septum pellucidum
(E) perforation of the lamina terminalis

1.5. Pick the *incorrect* pair:
(A) calcarine sulcus–visual cortex
(B) insula–primary auditory cortex
(C) postcentral gyrus–primary somesthetic cortex
(D) parahippocampal gyrus–primary olfactory area
(E) precentral gyrus–motor cortex

1.6. Cerebrospinal fluid (CFS) circulates from the lateral ventricle to the third ventricle via the:
(A) cerebral aqueduct
(B) foramen of Magendie
(C) central canal
(D) foramen of Monro
(E) foramina of Luschka

1.7. In a coronal section of the cerebrum at the level of the head of the caudate, the band of white matter separating the caudate nucleus from the putamen is the:
(A) external capsule
(B) genu of the internal capsule
(C) extreme capsule
(D) anterior limb of the internal capsule
(E) posterior limb of the internal capsule

1.8. The nuclear mass situated deep to the uncus is the:
(A) amygdala
(B) hippocampus
(C) globus pallidus
(D) putamen
(E) caudate nucleus

1.9. That part of the temporal lobe medial to the collateral sulcus is the:
(A) lingula
(B) inferior temporal gyrus
(C) parahippocampal gyrus
(D) occipitotemporal gyrus
(E) angulate gyrus

1.10. The lumbar cistern is a dilatation of:
(A) epidural space
(B) subarachnoid space
(C) subdural space
(D) space between intima pia and epipial layer
(E) central canal

1.11. The vertebral epidural space contains:
(A) cerebrospinal fluid
(B) internal vertebral venous plexus
(C) arachnoid trabeculae
(D) anterior and posterior spinal arteries
(E) potential space

For each numbered item, select the one heading most closely associated with it. Each lettered heading may be selected once, more than once, or not at all.

Questions 1.12–1.15

(A) Lateral ventricle
(B) Third ventricle
(C) Fourth ventricle
(D) Cerebral aqueduct
(E) Foramina of Luschka

1.12. Lamina terminalis

1.13. Septum pellucidum

1.14. Hypothalamus

1.15. Cerebellomedullary cistern

Questions 1.16–1.19

(A) Collateral sulcus
(B) Angular gyrus
(C) Gyrus rectus
(D) Cuneus
(E) Subcallosal gyrus

1.16. Parietal lobe

1.17. Temporal lobe

1.18. Occipital lobe

1.19. Olfactory tract

For each numbered item, select the letter designating the part in Fig. 1.1 which matches it correctly. A lettered part may be selected once, more than once, or not at all.

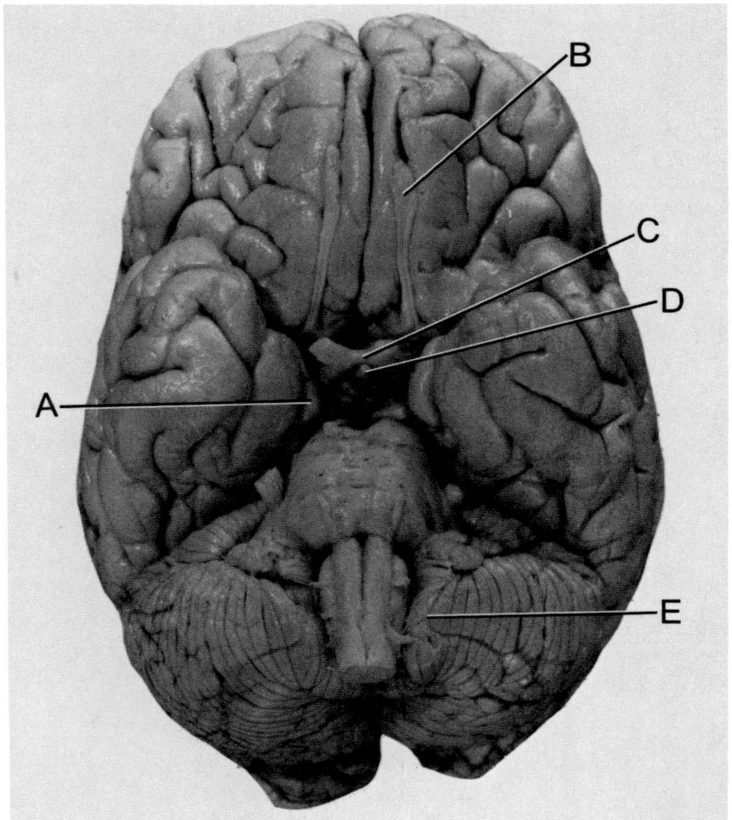

Figure 1.1. Ventral aspect of the cerebral hemispheres, brain stem, and cerebellum. (From D. E. Haines, *Neuroanatomy*, 1980; courtesy of Urban & Schwarzenberg, Baltimore.)

1.20. Partial decussation of sensory fibers

1.21. Receives primary sensory fibers associated with the phylogenetic oldest special sensory system

1.22. Herniation of this structure may produce a fixed dilated pupil

1.23. Herniation usually is fatal

For each numbered item, select the one heading most closely associated with it. Each lettered heading may be selected once, more than once, or not at all.

Questions 1.24–1.27

(A) Anterior horn lateral ventricle
(B) Posterior horn lateral ventricle
(C) Third ventricle
(D) Fourth ventricle
(E) Collateral trigone

1.24. Closely related to optic radiations and tapetum

1.25. Head of caudate nucleus forms lateral wall

1.26. Interventricular foramina

1.27. Choroid plexus emerges into subarachnoid space

Questions 1.28–1.31

(A) Choroid plexus capillaries
(B) Metabolic water
(C) Capillary bed of the brain
(D) Arachnoid villi
(E) Blood–CSF barrier

1.28. Formed by tight junctions of cuboidal epithelial cells

1.29. Produces about 70% of CSF with hydrostatic pressure

1.30. Serve as one-way valves when CSF pressure exceeds venous pressure

1.31. Enters the CSF when glucose is completely oxidized

For each numbered item, select the letter designating the part in Fig. 1.2 which matches it correctly. A lettered part may be selected once, more than once, or not at all.

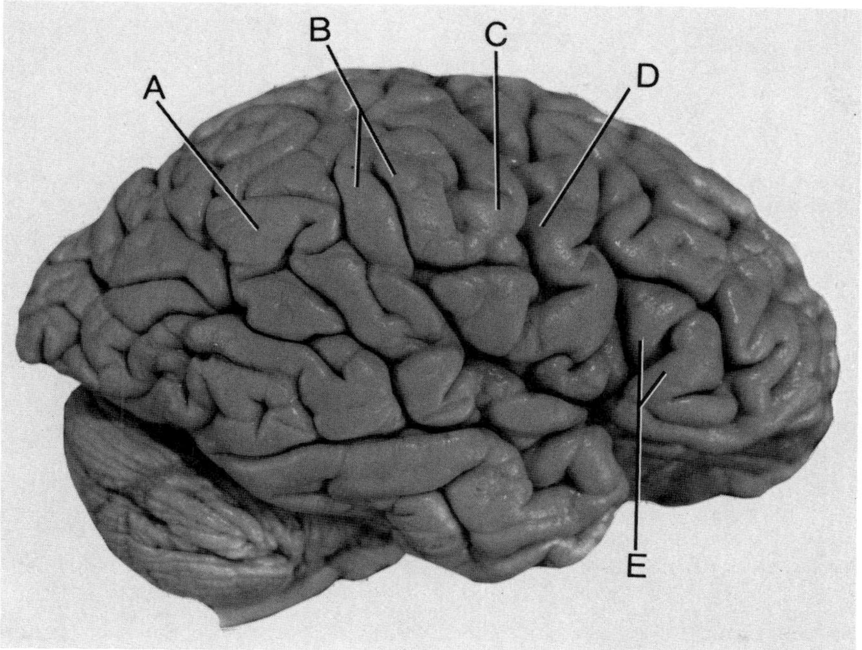

Figure 1.2. Lateral view of the right cerebral hemisphere and cerebellum. (From D. E. Haines, *Neuroanatomy*, 1983; courtesy of Urban & Schwarzenberg, Baltimore.)

1.32. Pars triangularis

1.33. Supramarginal gyrus

1.34. Angular gyrus

1.35. Primary somesthetic cortex

For each numbered item, select the one heading most closely associated with it. Each lettered heading may be selected once, more than once, or not at all.

Questions 1.36–1.39

(A) Epidural space
(B) Subarachnoid space
(C) Subdural space
(D) Fourth ventricle
(E) Lumbar cistern

1.36. Blockage of foramina will produce increased intracranial pressure

1.37. At spinal levels contains internal vertebral venous plexus

1.38. A potential space where venous blood may accumulate to produce a hematoma

1.39. Bleeding from branches of the middle meningeal artery may create this space

For each numbered item, select the letter designating the part in Fig. 1.3 which matches it correctly. A lettered part may be selected once, more than once, or not at all.

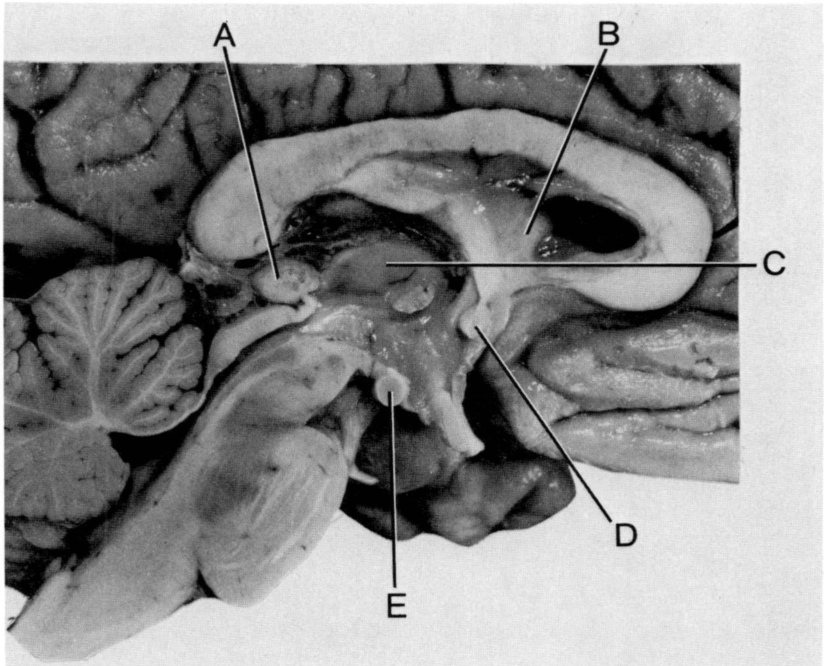

Figure 1.3. View of the medial surface of a hemisected brain. (From D. E. Haines, *Neuroanatomy*, 1983; courtesy of Urban & Schwarzenberg, Baltimore.)

1.40. Forms medial wall of anterior horn of lateral ventricle

1.41. Interconnects portions of the temporal lobe

1.42. Receives sensory inputs generated by somatic receptors

1.43. Concerned with circadian rhythms

For each numbered item, select the one heading most closely associated with it. Each lettered heading may be selected once, more than once, or not at all.

Questions 1.44–1.47

(A) Anterior limb internal capsule
(B) Posterior limb internal capsule
(C) Claustrum
(D) Extreme capsule
(E) Centrum semiovale

1.44. Lies immediate beneath insular cortex

1.45. Gray matter external to the lentiform nucleus

1.46. White matter containing commissural, association, and projection fibers identified in horizontal sections

1.47. Projection fibers situated between the head of the caudate nucleus and the putamen

Questions 1.48–1.51

(A) Transverse gyri of Heschl
(B) Tapetum
(C) Amygdaloid nuclear complex
(D) Visual radiations
(E) Gyrus rectus

1.48. Medial to olfactory bulb and tract

1.49. Corpus callosal fibers lateral to posterior horn of lateral ventricle

1.50. Afferent projections to calcarine cortex

1.51. Beneath cortex of uncus

For each numbered item, select the letter designating the part in Fig. 1.4 which matches it correctly. A lettered part may be selected once, more than once, or not at all.

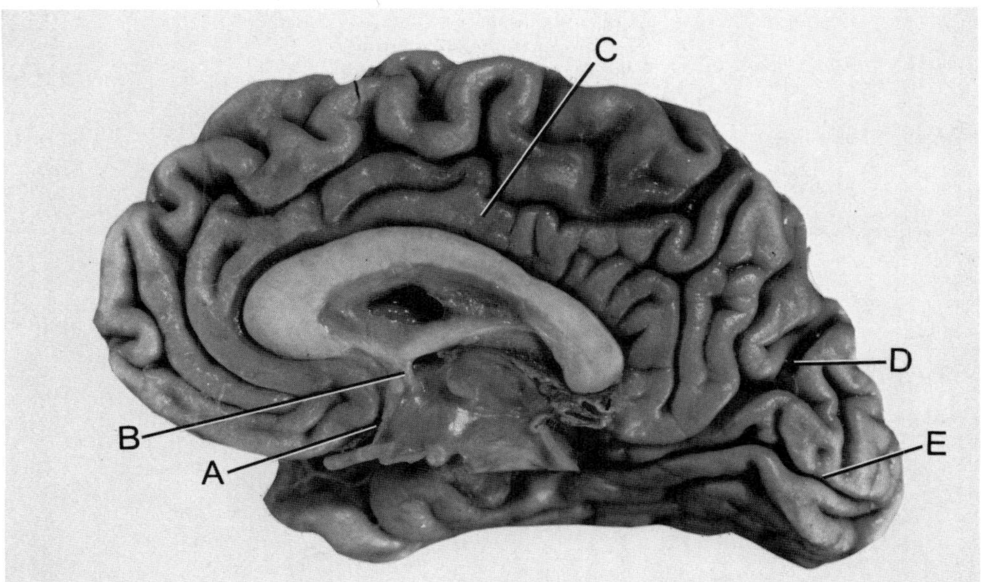

Figure 1.4. View of the medial surface of a midsagittal section of the cerebral hemisphere. (From D. E. Haines, *Neuroanatomy*, 1983; courtesy of Urban & Schwarzenberg, Baltimore.)

1.52. Separates the third ventricle and the subarachnoid space

1.53. Separate parietal and occipital lobes

1.54. Represent part of the contralateral visual field

1.55. Represents visceral functions and somatic functions related to visceral activities

For each numbered item, select the one heading most closely associated with it. Each lettered heading may be selected once, more than once, or not at all.

Questions 1.56–1.59

(A) Amygdala
(B) Hippocampal formation
(C) Head of caudate nucleus
(D) Thalamus
(E) Globus pallidus

1.56. Lies rostral to interventricular foramen

1.57. Lies rostral to inferior horn of lateral ventricle

1.58. Forms the lateral walls of the third ventricle

1.59. Situated between putamen and posterior limb of internal capsule

Questions 1.60–1.63

(A) Septum pellucidum
(B) Posterior commissure
(C) Hippocampal formation
(D) Anterior commissure
(E) Lamina terminalis

1.60. Surgical perforation could temporarily relieve noncommunicated hydrocephalus

1.61. Interconnects cortex of temporal lobe

1.62. Forms the medial wall of anterior horn of the lateral ventricle

1.63. Lies near choroidal fissure

For each numbered item, select the letter designating the part in Fig. 1.5 which matches it correctly. A lettered part may be selected once, more than once, or not at all.

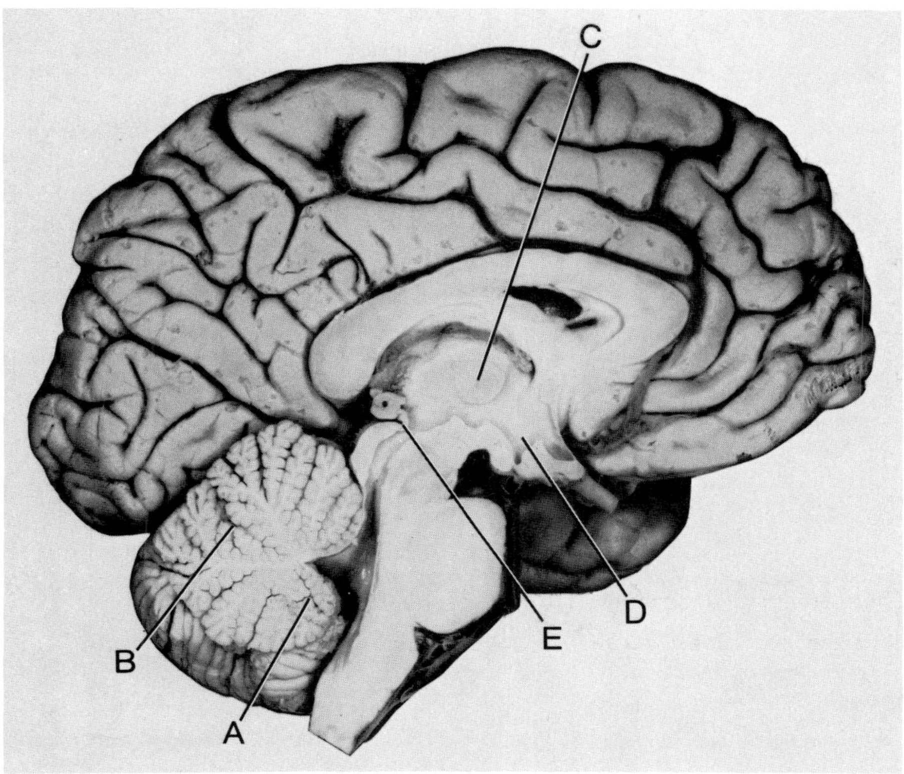

Figure 1.5. View of a midsagittal section of the brain. (From M. B. Carpenter and J. Sutin, *Human Neuroanatomy*, 1983; courtesy of Williams & Wilkins, Baltimore.)

1.64. Concerned with visceral, endocrine, and behavioral activities

1.65. Phylogenetically oldest cerebellar fissure

1.66. Separates paleocerebellum from neocerebellum

1.67. Marks the junction of mesencephalon and diencephalon

For each numbered item, indicate whether it is associated with

A only (A)
B only (B)
Both A and B (C)
Neither A or B (D)

Questions 1.68–1.72

(A) Choroid plexus
(B) Capillary bed of the brain
(C) Both
(D) Neither

1.68. Produces about 18% of the total CSF

1.69. Regulates the production and composition of the CSF

1.70. Produces CSF under a hydrostatic pressure

1.71. Controls pressure-dependent values in arachnoid villi

1.72. Transports hormone-releasing factors

Questions 1.73–1.76

(A) Blood-brain barrier
(B) Blood-CSF barrier
(C) Both
(D) Neither

1.73. Permits substances injected into CSF to enter the brain

1.74. Is permeable at circumventricular organs

1.75. Formed by tight junctions between choroid epithelial cells

1.76. Formed by tight junctions between endothelial cells of brain capillaries

Questions 1.77–1.80

(A) Dominant hemisphere
(B) Nondominant hemisphere
(C) Both
(D) Neither

1.77. Concerned with somesthetic perception

1.78. Particularly concerned with spatial concepts, recognition of faces and pictographic language

1.79. Processes spoken language and analytic functions

1.80. Controls the parameters of cardiovascular function

For each of the incomplete statements below, *one* or *more* of the completions given is correct. Choose answer:

(A) Only **1, 2,** and **3** are correct
(B) Only **1** and **3** are correct
(C) Only **2** and **4** are correct
(D) Only **4** is correct
(E) **All** are correct

1.81. Circulation of the cerebrospinal fluid in the CNS is dependent upon:
(1) unobstructed flow of CSF from the lateral ventricles to the cistern magna
(2) absorption of the CSF by the arachnoid granulations
(3) continuous CSF formation by the choroid plexus
(4) patency of the cavum septum pellucidum

1.82. The inferior parietal lobule is composed of:
(1) the postcentral gyrus
(2) the supramarginal gyrus
(3) the transverse gyri of Heschl
(4) the angular gyrus

1.83. The primary olfactory cortex:
(1) includes the uncus and part of the parahippocampal gyrus
(2) is not evident on the surface of the brain.
(3) receives the lateral olfactory stria
(4) includes temporal lobe cortex lateral to the collateral sulcus

1.84. Neural structures that follow the curvature of the lateral ventricle include:
(1) stria terminalis
(2) caudate nucleus
(3) fornix
(4) stria medullaris

1.85. In a patient with increased intracranial pressure due to an obstruction of the cerebral aqueduct, cerebrospinal fluid pressure could be reduced by:
(1) inserting a catheter in one lateral ventricle
(2) perforating the septum pellucidum
(3) perforating the lamina terminalis
(4) enlarging the foramen of Magendie

1.86. Fiber systems visible on the midsagittally sectioned brain include:
(1) corpus callosum
(2) anterior limb of the internal capsule
(3) fornix
(4) external capsule

1.87. Choroid plexus is present in:
(1) the interventricular foramina
(2) anterior horn of the lateral ventricle
(3) the posterior part of the fourth ventricle
(4) posterior horn of the lateral ventricle

1.88. The paracentral lobule:
(1) lies on the medial surface of the hemisphere
(2) has both somatic motor and sensory representation
(3) is concerned largely with the lower limb
(4) is part of the parietal lobe

1.89. The limbic lobe:
(1) consists of the subcallosal, cingulate and parahippocampal gyri
(2) is a synthetic lobe
(3) has predominantly representation of visceral functions
(4) represents somatic functions related to chewing, swallowing, and licking

1.90. The gyrus medial to the rhinal and collateral sulci:
(1) is a primary olfactory area
(2) has a medial protuberance known as the uncus
(3) overlies the amygdala
(4) is called the hippocampus

1.91. Following surgical section of the corpus callosum:
(1) sensory input received in the left hemisphere remains on that side
(2) the nondominant hemisphere is mute or dumb
(3) perceptive and cognitive activities in the two hemispheres are completely separate
(4) routine neurological examination would reveal no abnormality

1.92. The corpus callosum:
(1) connects homologous areas of the cerebral cortex by heavily myelinated fibers
(2) lies dorsal to fibers of the fornix
(3) conveys sensory information from one hemisphere to the other
(4) plays an essential role in speech

1.93. Following longitudinal surgical section of the corpus callosum in man:
(1) the nondominant hemisphere is mute
(2) analytic and mathematical functions are performed by the dominant hemisphere
(3) spatial concepts and recognition of faces are nondominant hemisphere functions
(4) the patient is unable to speak

Answers and Explanations*

1.1. **D** See p. 23
1.2. **D** See p. 30
1.3. **C** Fibers of the fornix originate from the hippocampal formation and from the subiculum. See p. 327
1.4. **B** Such a shunt would relieve the CSF pressure
1.5. **B**
1.6. **D** See pp. 13 and 35
1.7. **D** See p. 30
1.8. **A** See Figs. 2-16 and 12-8
1.9. **C** See p. 28; Fig. 2-8
1.10. **B** See p. 6; Fig. 1-7
1.11. **B** See p. 2; Fig. 14-3
1.12. **B** See Fig. 2-23
1.13. **A** See Figs. 2-22 and 2-23
1.14. **B** See Figs. 2-25 and 10-1
1.15. **E** See p. 6
1.16. **B** See Fig. 2-2
1.17. **A** See Fig. 2-8
1.18. **D** See Fig. 2-6
1.19. **C** See Fig. 2-7
1.20. **C** See Figs. 7-8 and 9-23
1.21. **B** See Figs. 12-1 and 12-2
1.22. **A** Uncal herniation at the tentorial notch puts pressure on, or stretches, the oculomotor nerve
1.23. **E** Herniation of the medulla and cerebellar tonsils in the foramen magnum
1.24. **B** See Figs. 2-9 and 9-24
1.25. **A** See Fig. 2-11
1.26. **C** See Fig. 2-18
1.27. **D** See Fig. 2-7
1.28. **E** See Fig. 1-15
1.29. **A** See p. 10
1.30. **D** See p. 7; Fig. 1-11
1.31. **B** See p. 12
1.32. **E** See Figs. 2-1 and 2-2
1.33. **B**
1.34. **A**
1.35. **C**
1.36. **D** Blockage of foramina of Luschka and Magendie
1.37. **A** See Fig. 14-3
1.38. **C**
1.39. **A** See Fig. 1-3
1.40. **B** Septum pellucidum
1.41. **D** Anterior commissure; see Fig. 2-12
1.42. **C** Dorsal thalamus
1.43. **A** Pineal gland; see pp. 225-226
1.44. **D** See Figs. 2-11 and 2-16
1.45. **C** See Figs. 2-11 and 2-16
1.46. **E** See Fig. 2-9
1.47. **A** See Fig. 2-11
1.48. **E** See Fig. 2-7
1.49. **B** See Fig. 2-9
1.50. **D** See Figs. 2-9, 9-23, and 9-24
1.51. **C** See Figs. 2-16 and 12-8
1.52. **A** Lamina terminalis, the membrane that closes the rostral neuropore
1.53. **D** Parieto-occipital sulcus
1.54. **E** Superior bank of the calcarine sulcus receives input via the lateral geniculate body from the superior quadrants of the retinae; these parts of the retinae subserve the inferior quadrants of contralateral visual field (see Fig. 9-23)
1.55. **C** Cingulate gyrus—part of the limbic lobe (see Fig. 12-17)
1.56. **C** See Fig. 2-11
1.57. **A** See Figs. 12-8 and 12-11
1.58. **D** See Figs. 2-23 and 2-25
1.59. **E** See Figs. 2-11 and 2-17

* All page numbers and illustration citations refer to Carpenter: CORE TEXT OF NEUROANATOMY, 3rd edition; © 1985, Williams & Wilkins.

1.60. **E** Lamina terminalis separates the rostral third ventricle from the subarachnoid space
1.61. **D** Anterior commissure
1.62. **A** See Figs. 2-22 and 2-23
1.63. **C** See Fig. 12-10
1.64. **D** Hypothalamus
1.65. **A** Posterolateral fissure
1.66. **B** Primary fissure
1.67. **E** Posterior commissure
1.68. **B** See p. 12
1.69. **A** See p. 12
1.70. **A** See p. 12
1.71. **D** See p. 7
1.72. **C** See p. 19
1.73. **D** Substances injected into the CSF enter the brain directly
1.74. **A** See p. 19
1.75. **B** See pp. 18–19; Fig. 1-15
1.76. **A** See pp. 14–17; Fig. 1-14
1.77. **C** Somesthetic perception involves both hemispheres equally
1.78. **B** See pp. 26 and 387–388
1.79. **A** See pp. 26 and 387–388
1.80. **D** Cardiovascular function is controlled by neurons in lower brain stem (see p. 126)
1.81. **A**
1.82. **C**
1.83. **B**
1.84. **A**
1.85. **B**
1.86. **B**
1.87. **B**
1.88. **A**
1.89. **E** See pp. 27–28; Fig. 12-17
1.90. **A**
1.91. **E** See p. 26
1.92. **A**
1.93. **A**

2

Spinal Cord

Questions

Select the one best answer

2.1. Spinal neurons classified as root cells are:
(A) internuncial neurons
(B) association neurons
(C) commissural neurons
(D) somatic and visceral efferent neurons
(E) neurons in laminae III and IV

2.2. All of the following symptoms would be seen in a lower motor neuron lesion, *except*:
(A) spasticity in the antigravity muscles
(B) muscular atrophy
(C) absent deep tendon reflexes
(D) muscular atonia
(E) fasciculations

2.3. Ascending spinal fibers conveying impulses related to painful and noxious stimuli:
(A) terminate in all parts of the ipsilateral ventral posterolateral (VPL) thalamic nucleus
(B) project to parts of the VPL, and bilaterally to the posterior thalamic nuclei and parts of the intralaminar thalamic nuclei
(C) project ipsilaterally to the posterior thalamic nuclei
(D) terminate mainly in the ventral posterolateral (VPL) and ventral posteromedial (VPM) thalamic nuclei
(E) project bilaterally to the intralaminar thalamic nuclei

2.4. A surgeon attempting to abolish pain in the pelvic region might make a lesion in the:
(A) cerebellum
(B) dorsal column nuclei
(C) posterior funiculus
(D) anterior part of the lateral funiculus
(E) anterior funiculus

2.5. Preganglionic parasympathetic neurons are located in:
(A) the intermediomedial cell column
(B) in sacral segments S2, S3, and S4
(C) in lumbar segments L2 through L4
(D) in all sacral segments
(E) in ganglia close to the structures they innervate

2.6. After sectioning several lumbar dorsal roots proximal to the spinal ganglia, the Nauta-Gygax stain might reveal degeneration in the:
(A) posterior spinocerebellar tract
(B) lateral spinothalamic tract
(C) fasciculus cuneatus
(D) anterior spinocerebellar tract
(E) fasciculus gracilis

2.7. The fibers of the lateral spinothalamic tract show the following segmental arrangement in the cervical spinal cord:
- (A) the posterior fibers conduct pain
- (B) the anterior fibers conduct thermal sense
- (C) the most lateral and posterior fibers represent the lowest portion of the body
- (D) the most medial and anterior fibers represent the lowest portions of the body
- (E) the most lateral and anterior fibers represent the upper extremity and neck region

2.8. Surgical section of the dorsal roots of C5 through C7 on one side between the dorsal root ganglia and the spinal cord would produce:
- (A) degeneration in all ascending tracts
- (B) ipsilateral degeneration in the fasciculus cuneatus and posterior spinocerebellar tracts and contralateral degeneration in the spinothalamic tracts and the anterior spinocerebellar tract
- (C) ipsilateral ascending and descending degeneration in the fasciculus cuneatus and the dorsolateral fasciculus
- (D) only ascending degeneration in the fasciculus cuneatus
- (E) ascending degeneration in the fasciculi gracilis and cuneatus

2.9. The lumbar cistern extends from:
- (A) L1 to L2
- (B) L2 to S2
- (C) L2 to S5
- (D) L4 to S2
- (E) T12 to S2

2.10. Descending autonomic fibers in the spinal cord are located in:
- (A) anterior funiculus
- (B) the posterior funiculus
- (C) the fasciculi proprii
- (D) the ventral part of the lateral funiculus
- (E) the dorsal half of the lateral funiculus

2.11. In the newborn the conus medullaris is located at the level of:
- (A) L5 vertebra
- (B) L2 vertebra
- (C) L3 vertebra
- (D) S3 vertebra
- (E) S5 vertebra

2.12. "Sensory dissociation" occurs with spinal lesions which selectively involve:
- (A) fibers of the posterior columns
- (B) spinocerebellar systems
- (C) fibers decussating in the ventral white commissure
- (D) the dorsal horn
- (E) spinal ganglia

2.13. In the Brown-Séquard syndrome:
- (A) pain, thermal, and tactile senses are lost contralaterally at slightly different levels below the lesion
- (B) discriminative tactile and kinesthetic senses are lost ipsilaterally below the level of the lesion
- (C) the tendon reflexes become exaggerated after a period of spinal shock
- (D) atrophy develops in muscles below the level of the lesion
- (E) the superficial abdominal and cremasteric reflexes are lost contralateral to the lesion

2.14. All of the statements concerning the posterior spinocerebellar tract are true, *except*:
- (A) conveys impulses from stretch, touch, and pressure receptors to the cerebellum
- (B) originates from cells of the dorsal nucleus of Clarke
- (C) does not extend below L3 spinal cord level
- (D) crosses at spinal levels in the anterior white commissure
- (E) enters the cerebellum by the inferior cerebellar peduncle

2.15. Horner's syndrome occurring in a patient with syringomyelia involving cervical spinal segments:
- (A) results from destruction of preganglionic neurons within the spinal cord
- (B) is due to involvement of descending autonomic fibers
- (C) is due to destruction of postganglionic fibers
- (D) results from involvement of reticular neurons in the medulla
- (E) is contralateral to the lesion

2.16. *Right* hemisection of the spinal cord at C4 would interrupt all of the following, *except*:
- (A) lateral corticospinal fibers from the left hemisphere
- (B) lateral spinothalamic fibers conveying pain and thermal sense from the left leg
- (C) fasciculus gracilis conveying kinesthetic sense from the left leg
- (D) posterior spinocerebellar input from the right side of the body
- (E) anterior corticospinal fibers from the right hemisphere

2.17. All of the following pairs match fiber tracts with cells of origin, *except*:
(A) medial lemniscus—nucleus cuneatus
(B) medullary reticulospinal tract—nucleus reticularis gigantocellularis
(C) vestibulospinal tract—medial vestibular nucleus
(D) spinothalamic tract—laminae I, IV, and V of the spinal cord
(E) posterior spinocerebellar tract—dorsal nucleus of Clarke

2.18. Lesions of the dorsal roots result in all of the following, *except*:
(A) loss of muscle tone
(B) anterograde degeneration in portions of the dorsal columns
(C) loss of myotatic reflexes
(D) anterograde degeneration in the lateral spinothalamic tract
(E) loss of cutaneous sensation in a restricted area

For each numbered item, select the one heading most closely associated with it. Each lettered heading may be selected once, more than once, or not at all.

Questions 2.19–2.22

(A) Dorsal nucleus of Clarke
(B) Cells in laminae I, IV, and V
(C) Substance P
(D) Dorsal root ganglia
(E) Intermediolateral cell column

2.19. Preganglionic sympathetic efferents

2.20. Spinothalamic tracts

2.21. Posterior spinocerebellar tract

2.22. Lamina I

Questions 2.23–2.26

(A) Locus ceruleus
(B) Posterior and paraventricular hypothalamic nuclei
(C) Nucleus raphe magnus
(D) Nucleus of solitary fasciculus
(E) Visceral nuclei of oculomotor complex

2.23. Project fibers ipsilaterally to intermediolateral cell column

2.24. Projects primarily crossed fibers to phrenic nerve nucleus and anterior horn cells in thoracic spinal segments

2.25. Is the source of noradrenergic fibers distributed in the spinal cord

2.26. Provides serotinergic projections to lamina I that inhibit substance P

Questions 2.27–2.30

(A) Facilitation of extensor muscle tone
(B) Facilitation of flexor muscle tone
(C) Inhibition of spasticity in antigravity muscles
(D) Excitation of alpha (α) motor neurons
(E) Inhibits both flexor and extensor muscle tone

2.27. Group Ia fibers

2.28. Medullary reticulospinal tract

2.29. Group Ib fibers

2.30. Vestibulospinal tract

For each numbered item, select the letter designating the part in Fig. 2.1 which matches it correctly. A lettered part may be selected once, more than once, or not at all.

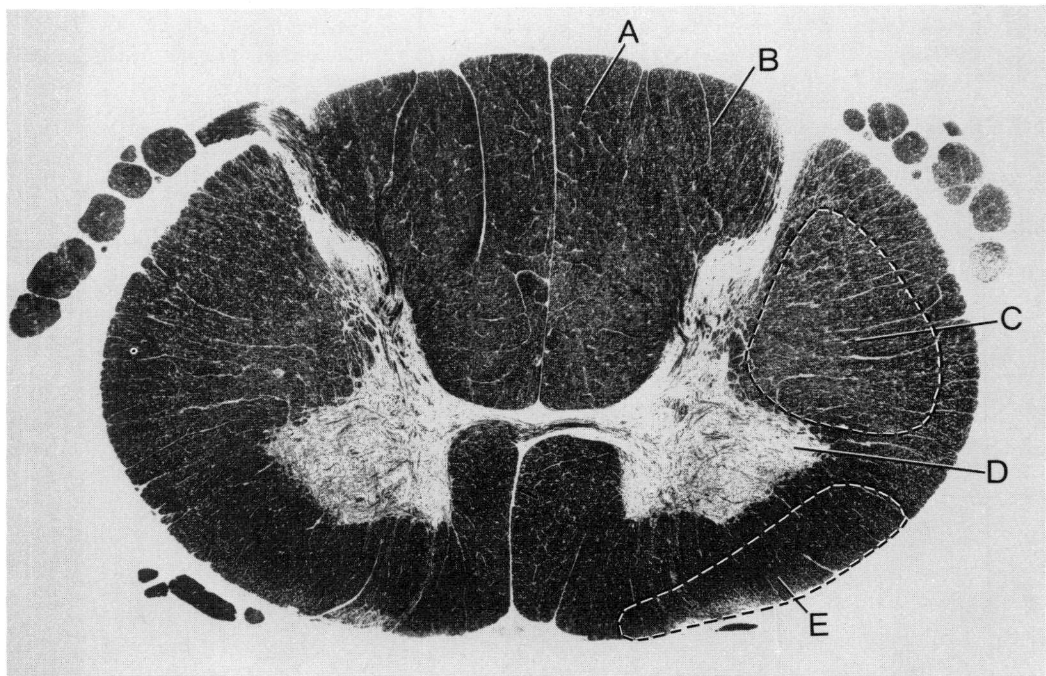

Figure 2.1. Transverse section of the spinal cord through the cervical enlargement. (From H. A. Riley, *Atlas of the Basal Ganglia, Brain Stem and Spinal Cord,* 1943; courtesy of Williams & Wilkins, Baltimore.

2.31. Region contains corticospinal and rubrospinal fibers

2.32. Region contains spinothalamic and vestibulospinal fibers

2.33. Projects to two distinct and separate medullary relay nuclei

2.34. Contains reticulospinal fibers terminating in Rexed's lamina IX

For each numbered item, select the one heading most closely associated with it. Each lettered heading may be selected once, more than once, or not at all.

Questions 2.35–2.38

(A) Mass reflex
(B) Reflex spinal sweating
(C) Clonus
(D) Spasticity
(E) Flaccidity

2.35. Self-perpetuating myotatic reflex

2.36. Independent of thermoregulator control

2.37. Bilateral triple flexion response produced by nonspecific stimuli

2.38. Most characteristic of lower motor neuron lesion

The lettered structures in Fig. 2.2 are correlated with a list of numbered phrases. For each numbered phrase, select the appropriate lettered structure.

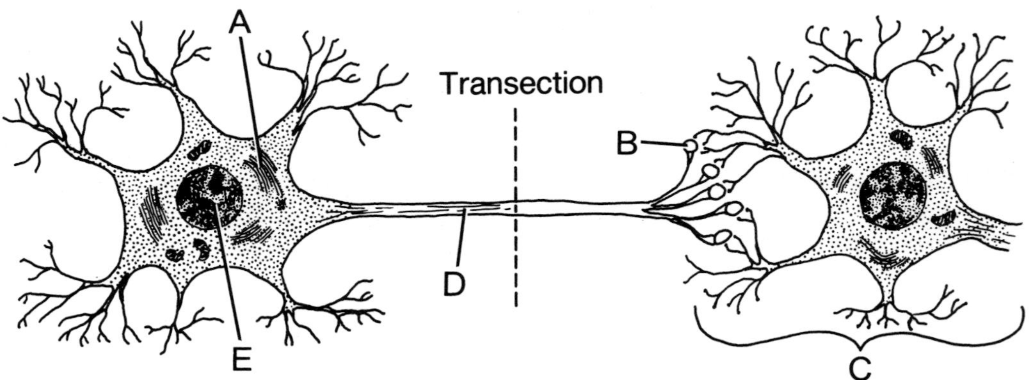

Figure 2.2. Schematic diagram of two neurons, one of which has the axon transected.

2.39. Will degenerate within a few days after the indicated injury.

2.40. May undergo chromatolysis after the indicated injury.

2.41. Axon sprouting is initiated from this portion of the neuron after the indicated injury

2.42. Degenerative changes are more likely to take place if the group of injured axons provided the sole input

For each numbered item, select the one heading most closely associated with it. Each lettered heading may be selected once, more than once, or not at all.

Questions 2.43–2.46

(A) Vestibulospinal tract
(B) Tectospinal tract
(C) Rubrospinal tract
(D) Corticospinal tract
(E) Reticulospinal tract

2.43. Facilitates ipsilateral flexor muscle reflexes

2.44. Terminates at cervical levels

2.45. Inhibits ipsilateral extensor reflexes

2.46. Modulates the activity of gamma (γ) motor neurons

For each numbered item, select the letter designating the part in Fig. 2.3 which matches it correctly. A lettered part may be selected once, more than once, or not at all.

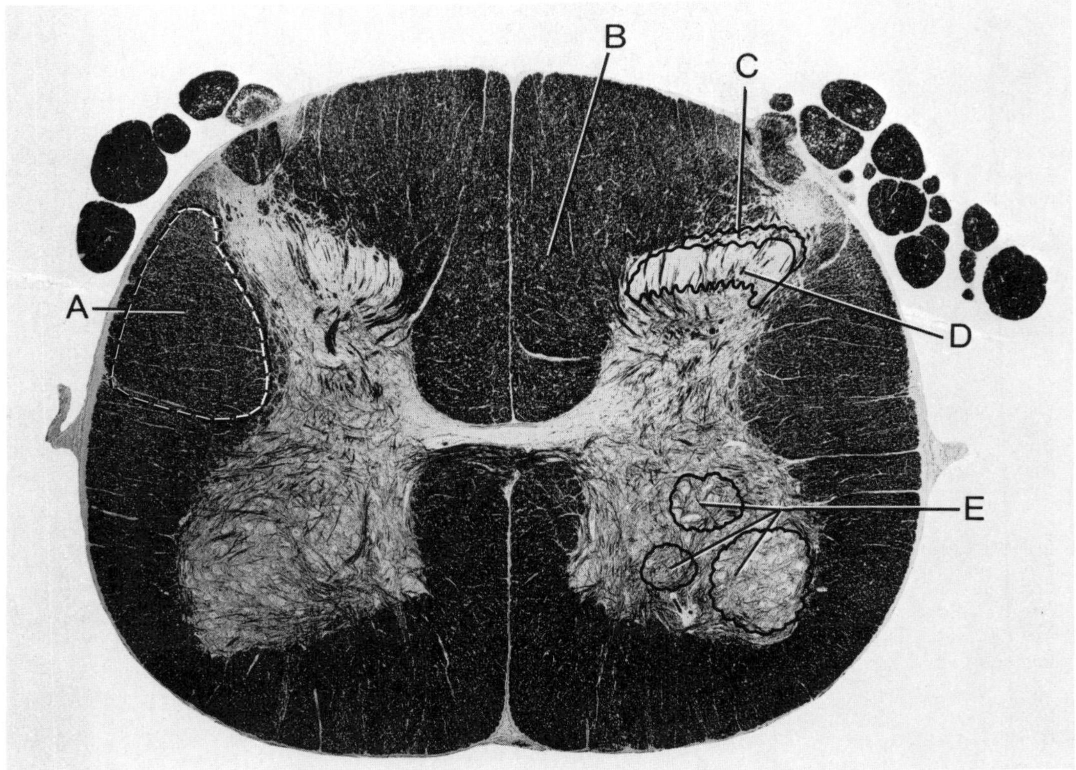

Figure 2.3. Photomicrograph of a transverse section of the lower lumbar spinal cord. (From H. A. Riley, *Atlas of the Basal Ganglia, Brain Stem and Spinal Cord*, 1943; courtesy of Williams & Wilkins, Baltimore.

2.47. Substantia gelatinosa (Rexed's lamina II)

2.48. Contains descending fibers most of which terminate in Rexed's lamina VII

2.49. Receive dorsal root fibers conveying impulses related to noxious stimuli

2.50. Contain α and γ motor neurons

For each numbered item, select the one heading most closely associated with it. Each lettered heading may be selected once, more than once, or not at all.

Questions 2.51–2.54

(A) Rubrospinal tract neurons
(B) Vestibulospinal tract neurons
(C) Medullary reticulospinal tract
(D) Hypothalamospinal tract
(E) Tectospinal tract

2.51. Neurons receive input from the cerebellar cortex

2.52. Neurons receive inputs from cerebral cortex and deep Cerebellar nuclei

2.53. Terminates upon cells of intermediolateral cell column

2.54. Coordinates head and eye movements

Questions 2.55–2.58

(A) Laminae I, IV, and V
(B) Lamina VII
(C) Lamina IX
(D) Laminae I and II
(E) Lamina VI

2.55. Present only in the enlargements of the spinal cord

2.56. Contains cells of the dorsal nucleus of Clarke and the intermediolateral cell column in thoracic segments

2.57. Contains α and γ motor neurons

2.58. Contains terminals of the corticospinal, rubrospinal, vestibulospinal, and reticulospinal tracts

For each numbered item, select the one lettered part most closely associated with it in Fig. 2.4. Each lettered part may be selected once, more than once, or not at all.

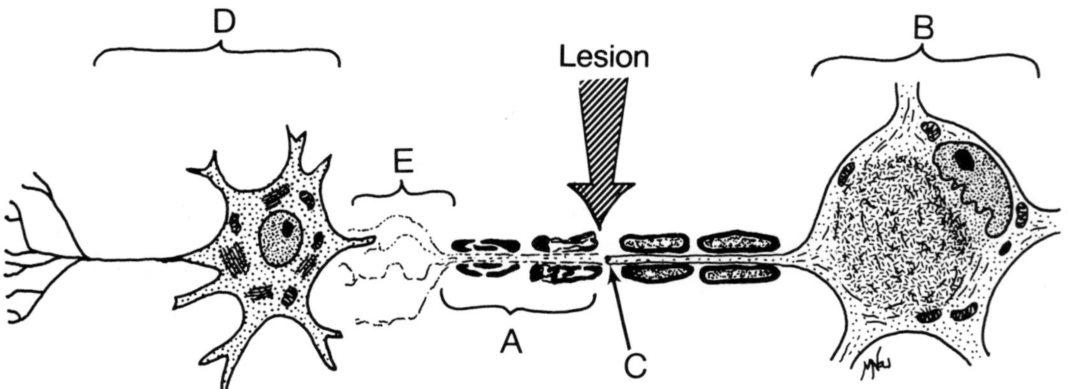

Figure 2.4. Schematic diagram of two neurons with lesion indicated by *large arrow.*

2.59. Degenerates within a few days after injury

2.60. Undergoing chromatolysis

2.61. After long period of time may undergo degeneration in some sensory systems

2.62. Wallerian degeneration

Each lettered part in Fig. 2.5 represents a lesion site. For each heading select the lettered part most closely associated with it. Each lettered part may be selected once, more than once, or not at all.

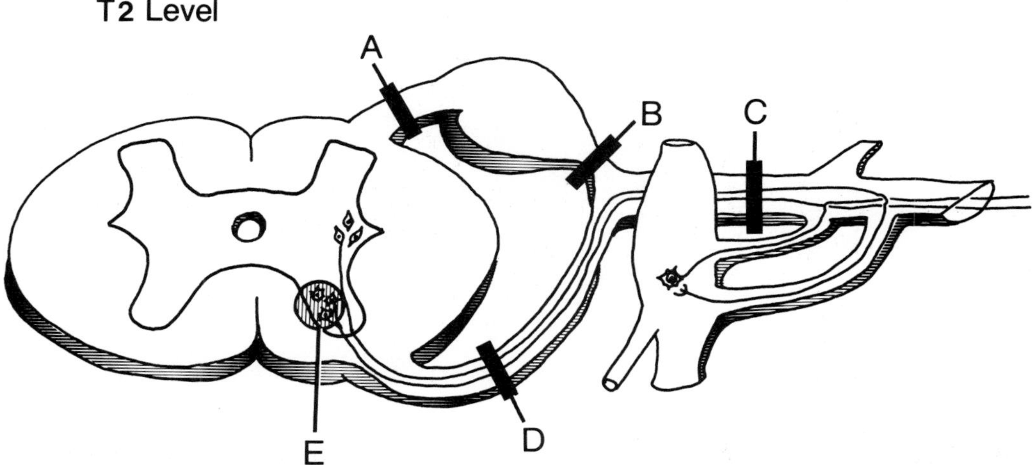

Figure 2.5. Schematic diagram of spinal cord, nerve roots, and peripheral ganglia.

2.63. Degeneration in posterior white column

2.64. Peripheral sensory and motor nerve degeneration

2.65. Degeneration in somatic motor and preganglionic sympathetic fibers

2.66. Only atrophy of somatic muscle

The lettered nuclei (*A*, *B*, *C*) in Fig 2.6 are correlated with a list of numbered phrases. For each numbered phrase, select the appropriate lettered nucleus (*A*, *B*, *C*)

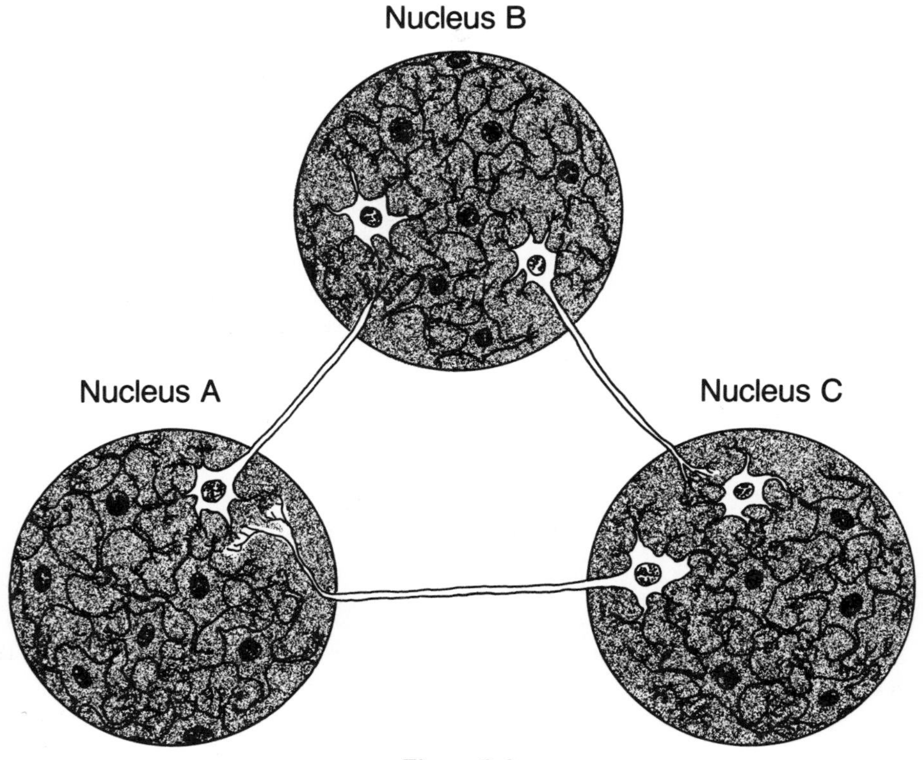

Figure 2.6

2.67. Horseradish peroxidase (HRP) injected into Nucleus B will label the cell bodies in

2.68. Tritiated amino acids injected into Nucleus C will in autoradiographs produce silver grains around the cell bodies and dendrites in

2.69. Horseradish peroxidase (HRP) may be taken up by the cell bodies of neurons in Nucleus B and transported to terminals in

2.70. If the neurons of Nucleus A are damaged (lesioned), anterograde terminal degeneration will be seen around the cell bodies and dendrites in

For each numbered item, indicate whether it is associated with

A only (A)
B only (B)
Both A and B (C)
Neither A or B (D)

Questions 2.71–2.75

(A) Muscle spindle
(B) Golgi tendon organ
(C) Both
(D) Neither

2.71. Clonus

2.72. Myotatic reflex

2.73. Mass reflex

2.74. Inverse myotatic reflex

2.75. Afferents to gamma motor neurons

Questions 2.76–2.79

(A) Fasciculus gracilis
(B) Fasciculus cuneatus
(C) Both
(D) Neither

2.76. Contain primary afferent fibers

2.77. Associated with lower extremity

2.78. Convey impulses associated with two-point discrimination and kinesthesis

2.79. Horseradish peroxidase (HRP) injected into spinal ganglion at T5 would accumulate in granules within cells of a dorsal column nucleus

For each lettered part in the immunoreactive section shown in Fig. 2.7, indicate whether it is associated with

A only (A)
B only (B)
Both A and B (C)
Neither A nor B (D)

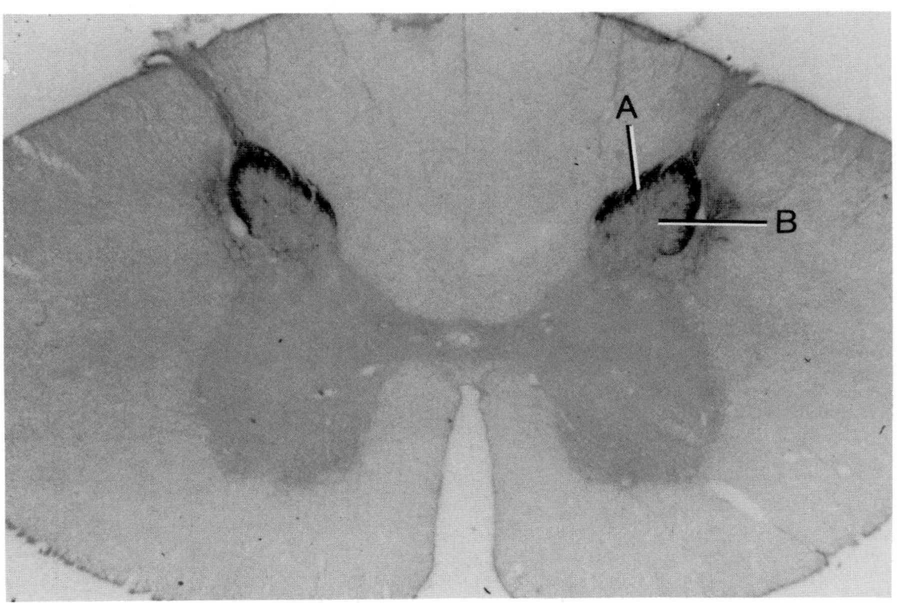

Figure 2.7. Photomicrograph of immunoreacted section of the spinal cord. (From M. B. Carpenter and J. Sutin, *Human Neuroanatomy*, 1983; courtesy of Williams & Wilkins, Baltimore.)

2.80. Receives fibers concerned with non-nociceptive stimuli

2.81. Receives fibers from dorsal root ganglion cells

2.82. Receives fibers from dorsal root ganglion cells having substance P as their neurotransmitter

2.83. Enkephalin may inhibit excitation produced by nociceptive stimuli

For each lettered transverse section in Fig. 2.8, indicate whether it is associated with

A only (A)
B only (B)
Both A and B (C)
Neither A nor B (D)

2.84. Contains preganglionic autonomic neurons

2.85. Contains α motor neurons innervating appendicular musculature

2.86. Contains fibers of both anterior and posterior spinocerebellar tracts

2.87. Contains the smallest number of corticospinal fibers

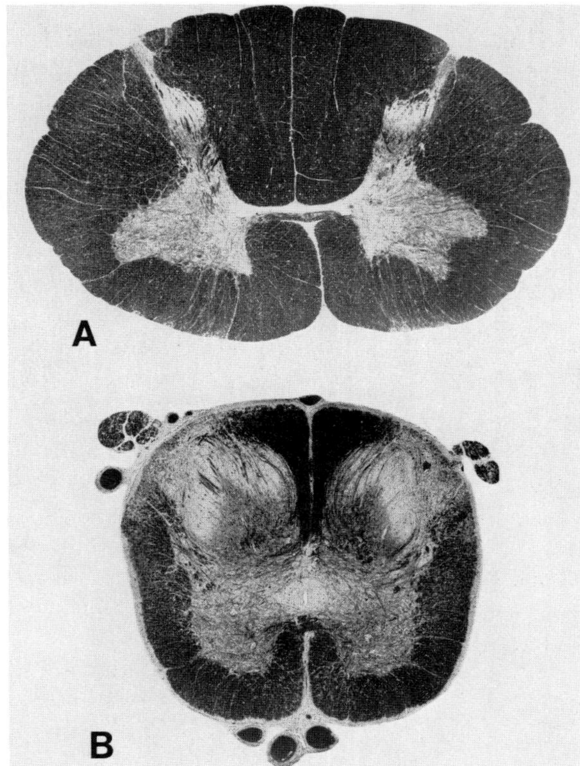

Figure 2.8. Two transverse Weigert-stained sections of the spinal cord at different levels. (From H. A. Riley, *Atlas of the Basal Ganglia, Brain Stem and Spinal Cord*, 1943; courtesy of Williams & Wilkins, Baltimore.)

For each lettered transverse section in Fig. 2.9, indicate whether it is associated with

A only (A)
B only (B)
Both A and B (C)
Neither A nor B (D)

2.88. The most caudal of these sections

2.89. Contains cells of origin of posterior spinocerebellar tract

2.90. Contains ascending branches of dorsal root ganglion cells

2.91. Contains preganglionic sympathetic neurons

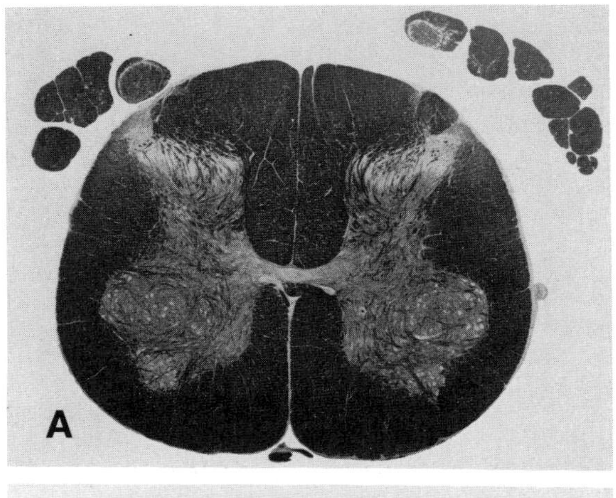

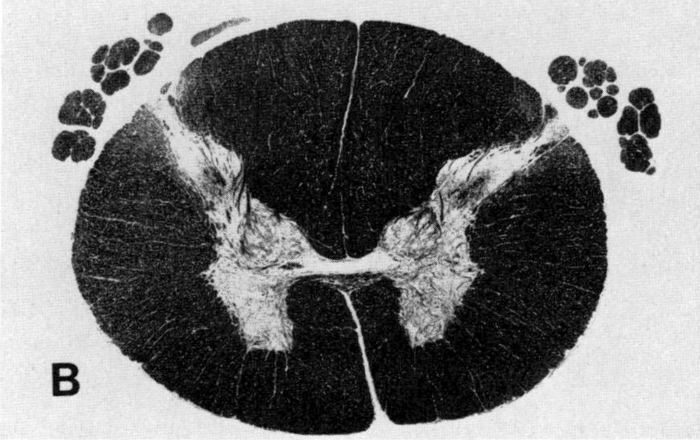

Figure 2.9. Two transverse Weigert-stained sections of the spinal cord at different levels. (From H. A. Riley, *Atlas of the Basal Ganglia, Brain Stem and Spinal Cord*, 1943; courtesy of Williams & Wilkins, Baltimore.)

For each of the incomplete statements below, *one* or *more* of the completions given is correct. Choose answer:

(A) Only **1, 2,** and **3** are correct
(B) Only **1** and **3** are correct
(C) Only **2** and **4** are correct
(D) Only **4** is correct
(E) **All** are correct

2.92. Tracts which descend in the ventral funiculus or sulcomarginal area of the spinal cord, include the:
(1) vestibulospinal
(2) pontine reticulospinal
(3) interstitiospinal
(4) rubrospinal

2.93. Decussations in the anterior white commissure, include:
(1) posterior spinocerebellar tract
(2) anterior and lateral spinothalamic tracts
(3) vestibulospinal tract
(4) anterior spinocerebellar tract

2.94. A Horner's syndrome may result from lesions:
(1) involving the intermediolateral cell column at T1
(2) in the brain stem involving descending pathways from the hypothalamus
(3) in the cervical spinal cord involving ventral portions of the lateral funiculus
(4) in the superior cervical ganglion

2.95. The substantia gelatinosa:
(1) is equivalent to Rexed's lamina I
(2) is best developed in cervical and lumbar enlargements
(3) gives rise to the posterior spinocerebellar tract
(4) is similar in function and appearance to the spinal trigeminal nucleus

2.96. Damage to the ventral roots of spinal nerves T5–L2 may produce:
(1) retrograde cell changes in the anterior horn cells of spinal cord segments T5–L2
(2) retrograde cell changes in the intermediolateral cell column of thoracic spinal cord segments
(3) demyelination of axons in spinal nerves T5–L2
(4) retrograde cell changes in the dorsal nucleus of Clarke at these spinal cord levels (T5–L2)

2.97. The posteromarginal nucleus of the dorsal horn:
(1) receives primary dorsal root afferents utilizing substance P as a neurotransmitter
(2) receives short axons from the substantia gelatinosa
(3) is rich in opiate receptors thought to mediate analgesia effects.
(4) has short axons that monosynaptically excite α motor neurons

2.98. Sensory modalities reaching the conscious sphere are transmitted via:
(1) fasciculus gracilis and cuneatus
(2) spino-olivary pathways
(3) anterior and lateral spinothalamic tracts
(4) anterior and posterior spinocerebellar tracts

2.99. Spinal projections from the nucleus raphe magnus:
(1) are mainly crossed
(2) terminate bilaterally in lamina I
(3) descend only in the ventral funiculus
(4) suppress transmission of signals related to painful stimuli

2.100. Following severance of an axon relatively close to the neuronal soma:
(1) the soma imbibes water and the nucleus becomes eccentric
(2) Nissl bodies become fragmented and dispersed
(3) the distal part of the axon undergoes Wallerian degeneration
(4) protein synthesis in the soma is inhibited

2.101. Surgical section of dorsal roots C5 through T1 produces:
(1) degeneration in all ascending spinal tracts
(2) ascending long tract degeneration only in the ipsilateral fasciculus cuneatus
(3) ascending degeneration in the ipsilateral fasciculus cuneatus and posterior spinocerebellar tracts and the contralateral spinothalamic tracts
(4) terminal degeneration in ipsilateral cuneate and accessory cuneate nuclei

2.102. The myotatic reflex involves:
(1) the muscle spindle
(2) the Golgi tendon organ
(3) group Ia muscle afferents
(4) group Ib muscle afferents

2.103. In the inverse myotatic reflex, evoked by powerful flexion or extension of a spastic limb:
(1) impulses arising from the Golgi tendon organ predominate over those from the muscle spindle
(2) at least two synapses are involved
(3) there is inhibition of α motor neurons
(4) there is facilitation of γ motor neurons

2.104. Spinal and medullary relay nuclei receiving group Ia afferent fibers are:
(1) dorsal nucleus of Clarke
(2) cells of Rexed's lamina IX
(3) accessory cuneate nucleus
(4) Rexed's lamina I

2.105. Spinal pathways conveying impulses from stretch receptors in the lower extremity:
(1) are the spinothalamic tracts
(2) project to the cerebellar vermis
(3) consist of numerous short relays
(4) largely compose the anterior and posterior spinocerebellar tracts

2.106. A crush injury of the upper lumbar spinal cord would produce degeneration in the:
(1) fasciculus cuneatus
(2) posterior spinocerebellar tract
(3) cuneocerebellar tract
(4) fasciculus gracilis

2.107. The dorsal column system:
(1) transmits pain information
(2) consists of axons from neurons in Clarke's column
(3) transmits thermal sense
(4) consists of ascending collaterals of tactile and kinesthetic primary afferents

2.108. Myotatic reflexes are reduced or abolished for involved spinal cord segments following:
(1) dorsal rhizotomy
(2) poliomyelitis
(3) lesions of the ventral root
(4) tabes dorsalis

2.109. Structures found in the gray matter at the T12 spinal segment include the:
(1) nucleus dorsalis of Clarke
(2) intermediolateral nucleus
(3) medial motoneuronal group
(4) lateral (distal) motoneuronal groups

2.110. Syringomyelia in its early stage is characterized by:
(1) loss of pain sensation bilaterally
(2) loss of two-point tactile sensation
(3) loss of thermal sense
(4) loss of kinesthesis

2.111. Large caliber dorsal root fibers:
(1) enter on the medial side of the dorsal horn
(2) comprise the tract of Lissauer
(3) give off collaterals which ascend and descend in the dorsal funiculi
(4) convey pain and thermal sense

2.112. The spinothalamic (anterolateral) system:
(1) conveys pain, temperature, and light touch
(2) crosses in the anterior white commissure
(3) is somatotopically organized
(4) contains fibers that terminate in the ventral posterolateral (VPLc), intralaminar and posterior thalamic nuclei

2.113. Sensory dissociation:
(1) occurs bilaterally and fairly symmetrically in syringomyelia
(2) usually preserves pain and the thermal sense
(3) results from lesions near the central canal that destroy the anterior white commissure
(4) may occur in leprosy

2.114. In the myotatic reflex:
(1) the receptor excited by the stimulus is the Golgi tendon organ
(2) the excited receptor element is the muscle spindle
(3) afferent volleys excite γ motor neurons
(4) afferent input excites α motor neurons monosynaptically

2.115. Weakness, fasciculations and atrophy of the small intrinsic muscles of the hands without sensory loss suggests a pathological process involving:

(1) α motor neurons
(2) γ motor neurons
(3) C8, T1 spinal levels
(4) C5, C6 spinal levels

2.116. A somatotopic organization is characteristic of:

(1) the lateral spinothalamic tract
(2) the rubrospinal tract
(3) the posterior columns
(4) the lateral corticospinal tract

2.117. Reticulospinal tracts:

(1) arise from the medullary and pontine reticular formation
(2) exhibit only facilitory influences for reflex activity
(3) are primarily uncrossed
(4) distribute fibers chiefly to lamina IX of the spinal gray

2.118. Descending autonomic fiber systems projecting to spinal levels arise from:

(1) locus ceruleus
(2) hypothalamus
(3) nuclei of the solitary fasciculus
(4) vestibular nuclei

2.119. Selective surgical section of the fasciculus gracilis and cuneatus at C5 would:

(1) abolish the myotatic reflexes in the lower extremities
(2) abolish discriminative tactile and kinesthetic sense below C5
(3) diminish muscle tone in the legs
(4) have no effect upon myotatic reflexes in the lower limbs

2.120. Spinal shock in man:

(1) lasts 1–6 weeks
(2) is associated with absences of all neural activity below the level of the lesion
(3) occurs only with spinal cord transection
(4) is sometimes seen with unilateral spinal cord lesions

2.121. Surgical section of dorsal roots C5 through T1:

(1) reduces muscle tone in the upper extremity
(2) abolishes myotatic (deep tendon) relfexes in most of the ipsilateral upper extremity
(3) eliminates most cutaneous sensation in C6, C7, and C8 dermatomes
(4) abolishes sensation in the upper extremity

2.122. The spinal part of the accessory nerve:

(1) emerges from the lateral surface of the spinal cord
(2) passes rostrally dorsal to the denticulate ligaments
(3) supplies the sternocleidomastoid and upper portions of the trapezius muscles
(4) arises from the upper 5 (or 6) cervical spinal segments

2.123. Pseudounipolar neurons of dorsal root ganglia:

(1) receive no axosomatic synapses
(2) may have extremely long axons
(3) provide both somatic and visceral sensory innervation
(4) establish afferent limbs of reflex arcs

Answers and Explanations*

2.1. **D** Fibers of root cells emerge via the ventral root (see p. 57)

2.2. **A** See p. 95

2.3. **B** See p. 80

2.4. **D** Anterolateral cordotomy interrupts fibers of the spinothalamic tracts

2.5. **B** See p. 67

2.6. **E** Fibers ascending in the fasciculus gracilis represent branches of lumbar spinal ganglia. All other tracts ascending from the lumbar spinal cord arise from intrinsic spinal neurons

2.7. **D**

2.8. **C** Fibers in these tracts arise from cervical spinal ganglia

2.9. **B** See p. 6

2.10. **D**

2.11. **C** See p. 52

2.12. **C** Syringomyelia presents a "sensory dissociation" in which pain and thermal sense are lost, but other modalities are preserved

2.13. **B** Although pain and thermal sense are lost contralaterally below the level of the lesion, tactile sense remains on that side. The contralateral posterior remains intact

2.14. **D** The posterior spinocerebellar tract is uncrossed

2.15. **B**

2.16. **C** Fasciculus gracilis is uncrossed

2.17. **C** The vestibulospinal tract arises from the lateral vestibular nucleus

2.18. **D** Degeneration here does not pass beyond the first synapse

2.19. **E**

2.20. **B** See pp. 77–81

2.21. **A** See p. 81

2.22. **C** See p. 72; Fig. 3-21

2.23. **B** See p. 95; Fig. 4-15

2.24. **D**

2.25. **A**

2.26. **C** See p. 114

2.27. **D** Afferents from muscle spindles have an excitatory action on alpha motor neurons

2.28. **E** See p. 94

2.29. **C** Afferents from Golgi tendon organs have a disynaptic inhibitory action on alpha motor neurons

2.30. **A** See p. 91

2.31. **C**

2.32. **E**

2.33. **B** Fasciculus cuneatus projects to the ipsilateral cuneate and accessory cuneate nuclei

2.34. **E**

2.35. **C** See p. 99

2.36. **B** Occur below the level of spinal transection

2.37. **A** See p. 99

2.38. **E** See p. 95

2.39. **B** Terminal boutons

2.40. **A** Retrograde chromatolysis

2.41. **D** Especial at node of Ranvier

2.42. **C** Transneuronal degeneration such as is seen in the lateral geniculate body

2.43. **C** In spinal cord facilitates ipsilateral flexor muscles

2.44. **B** See p. 89

2.45. **C** See p. 90

2.46. **E** See p. 93

2.47. **D**

2.48. **A**

2.49. **C** Rexed's lamina I

* All page numbers and illustration citations refer to Carpenter: CORE TEXT OF NEUROANATOMY, 3rd edition; © 1985, Williams & Wilkins.

2.50. **E** Rexed's lamina IX

2.51. **B** Cerebellovestibular fibers from anterior lobe vermis (see p. 216) and fibers from fastigial nuclei

2.52. **A** Corticorubral fibers and projections from emboliform nucleus (see Fig. 8-14)

2.53. **D** See Fig. 4-15

2.54. **E** See pp. 89 and 178-179

2.55. **E** See p. 65

2.56. **B** See p. 66

2.57. **C** See p. 68

2.58. **B**

2.59. **E** Terminal fibers and boutons

2.60. **B** Retrograde chromatolysis

2.61. **D** Transneuronal degeneration

2.62. **A** Degeneration distal to lesion

2.63. **A** Lesion at *B* produces degeneration in peripheral somatic and visceral afferent fibers and chromatolysis in ganglion cells, but no central degeneration

2.64. **C** Lesion of mixed spinal nerve

2.65. **D**

2.66. **E** Lesion in part of anterior horn

2.67. **A** Retrograde transport of HRP to cell somata

2.68. **A** Anterograde transport of protein precursors

2.69. **C** Anterograde transport of HRP from cell somata to fiber terminals

2.70. **B** Anterograde degeneration

2.71. **A** Extreme exaggeration of myotatic reflex

2.72. **A** Receptor is muscle spindle

2.73. **D** Involves reflexor reflex afferents

2.74. **B** Sudden loss of spasticity with power stretch of the muscle due to disynaptic inhibition evoked by stimulation of Golgi tendon organ

2.75. **D** Neither supplies afferents to γ motor neurons

2.76. **C**

2.77. **A**

2.78. **C**

2.79. **D** HRP is not transported transneuronally

2.80. **B** Rexed's lamina II

2.81. **C** See pp. 69–72

2.82. **A** Rexed's lamina I

2.83. **A** Rexed's lamina I

2.84. **D** A is cervical enlargement and B is coccygeal

2.85. **A** Only *A*

2.86. **A** Only *A*

2.87. **B** Most of the corticospinal fibers have been given off at segmental levels rostral to coccygeal segments

2.88. **A** Sacral 5 segment

2.89. **B** Dorsal nucleus of Clarke (nucleus thoracicus)

2.90. **C** Contained in fasciculus gracilis

2.91. **B** Lumbar 1 contains cells of intermediolateral cell column

2.92. **A**

2.93. **C**

2.94. **E** All are correct

2.95. **C** See p. 63

2.96. **A**

2.97. **B** See p. 72

2.98. **B**

2.99. **C** See p. 114

2.100. **A**

2.101. **C**

2.102. **B** See p. 72

2.103. **A** This is the basis for the collapse of spasticity, if powerful passive flexion or extension is applied. It is also referred to as the lengthening reaction, which protects the muscle from injury by overstretching

2.104. **A** Group Ia fibers passing to lamina IX are involved in the myotatic reflex; fibers passing to the dorsal nucleus of Clarke and the accessory cuneate nucleus are parts of cerebellar afferent systems

2.105. **C**

2.106. **C**

2.107. **D**

2.108. **E**

2.109. **A** T12 does not supply appendicular musculature

2.110. **B** If the syringx is small, it will involve primarily the fibers crossing in the ventral white commissure

2.111. **B**

2.112. **E**

2.113. B

2.114. C See pp. 72-73

2.115. B

2.116. A In the spinal cord there is little somatotopical organization in the corticospinal tract

2.117. B See pp. 91-94

2.118. A See p. 95; Fig. 4-15

2.119. C The reflex arcs caudal to the lesion would be intact

2.120. A See p. 99

2.121. A See pp. 98–99

2.122. E See p. 121

2.123. E See pp. 69-73

3

Medulla

Questions

Select the one best answer

3.1. Select the *discordant* pair:
- (A) accessory cuneate nucleus-Clarke's column
- (B) inferior olive-cerebellar relay
- (C) nucleus ambiguus-muscles of the pharynx and larynx
- (D) medial longitudinal fasciculus (MLF)-dorsal column axons
- (E) tractus solitarius-visceral sensation

3.2. In a Weigert-stained section of the rostral medulla, the large dark mass capped by the dorsal and ventral cochlear nuclei is the:
- (A) tractus solitarius
- (B) medial lemniscus
- (C) superior cerebellar peduncle
- (D) inferior olive
- (E) inferior cerebellar peduncle

3.3. A lesion involving the nucleus ambiguus could produce all of the following, *except*:
- (A) paralysis of the palate
- (B) paralysis of the pharynx
- (C) hoarseness of the voice
- (D) paralysis of lower esophagus
- (E) paralysis of upper esophagus

3.4. Stimulating the dorsal motor nucleus of the vagus nerve might elicit each of the following, *except*:
- (A) contraction of the bladder
- (B) gastrointestinal peristalsis
- (C) bronchial constriction
- (D) contraction of the gall bladder
- (E) bradycardia

3.5. A patient with loss of pain and thermal sense on one side of the face and on the opposite side of the body has sustained a lesion in:
- (A) the postcentral gyrus
- (B) the pontine tegmentum
- (C) the dorsolateral quadrant of the medulla
- (D) the substantia gelatinosa of C1
- (E) the midbrain tegmentum

3.6. The most immediate threat to survival associated with bilateral lesions of the vagus nerve is:
- (A) loss of vagal respiratory reflexes
- (B) complete laryngeal paralysis
- (C) cardiac acceleration
- (D) loss of the gag reflex and inability to swallow
- (E) regurgitation and aspiration of liquids

3.7. Trigeminal tractotomy (i.e., section of the spinal trigeminal tract) performed at the level of the obex in a patient with trigeminal neuralgia:
- (A) will abolish pain and thermal sense in the ipsilateral half of the face with minimal impairment of tactile sense
- (B) will eliminate pain and thermal sense ipsilaterally only in the mandibular distribution of the trigeminal nerve
- (C) will eliminate pain in the face ipsilaterally and abolish the corneal reflex
- (D) will abolish all sensation in the trigeminal distribution
- (E) will eliminate the jaw jerk (myotatic reflex)

3.8. Group Ia fibers in the upper roots of the brachial plexus, conveying impulses to the cerebellum, synapse in:
(A) Clarke's column
(B) lamina VII
(C) the cuneate nucleus
(D) the accessory cuneate nucleus
(E) none of these

3.9. Cortical influences upon the hypoglossal motor neurons are conveyed:
(A) primarily by corticoreticular fibers
(B) bilaterally only by direct corticobulbar fibers
(C) by crossed corticobulbar fibers that pass directly to hypoglossal nucleus
(D) bilaterally by direct corticobulbar fibers and indirectly by corticoreticular fibers transmitting impulses to reticular neurons
(E) via the cerebellum and reticular formation

3.10. The carotid sinus reflex:
(A) involves chemoreceptors in the carotid body
(B) involves the glossopharyngeal afferents and efferent fibers from the dorsal motor nucleus of the vagus
(C) involves afferent impulses from the baroreceptor which produce an elevation of arterial blood pressure
(D) is mediated entirely by the vagus nerve
(E) is mediated only by the glosspharyngeal nerve

3.11. The glossopharyngeal nerve:
(A) conveys taste sensation from the anterior ⅔ of the tongue
(B) conveys taste sensation from the posterior ⅓ of the tongue
(C) conveys taste and general sensation from the posterior ⅓ of the tongue
(D) is concerned almost exclusively with parasympathetic innervation of the salivary glands
(E) innervates the constrictor muscles of the pharynx

3.12. The medullary equivalent of dorsolateral fasciculus of Lissauer is the:
(A) fasciculus solitarius
(B) spinal trigeminal tract
(C) internal arcuate fibers
(D) inferior olivary complex
(E) stria medullaris of medulla

3.13. Internal arcuate fibers in the lower medulla:
(A) arise from the arcuate nucleus
(B) arise from the posterior column nuclei and the accessory cuneate nucleus
(C) conveys impulses from stretch receptors to the cerebellum
(D) give collaterals to the reticular formation
(E) form the contralateral medial lemniscus

3.14. General somatic efferent fibers are carried in all of the following cranial nerves, *except*:
(A) VI
(B) V
(C) XII
(D) III
(E) IV

3.15. Brain stem nuclei which receive general somatic afferent fibers include the:
(A) solitary nuclei
(B) vestibular nuclei
(C) trigeminal nuclear complex
(D) cochlear nuclei
(E) dorsal motor nucleus and nucleus ambiguus

3.16. Lesions in which following will *not* produce a Horner's syndrome:
(A) superior cervical ganglion
(B) posterior hypothalamus
(C) intermediolateral cell column in upper thoracic spinal segments
(D) medullary raphe nuclei
(E) ventral quadrant of cervical spinal cord

3.17. The medullary reticular formation projects fibers to:
(A) cerebellum
(B) all spinal levels
(C) motor and sensory cranial nerve nuclei
(D) higher levels of the brain stem
(E) all of the above

3.18. Pseudobulbar palsy:
(A) is characterized by loss of emotional control and involvement of lower motor neurons in the brain stem
(B) is a syndrome due to bilateral, diffuse involvement of corticobulbar fiber systems
(C) involves pathways to sensory relay nuclei in the lower brain stem
(D) involves multiple descending systems on one side of the brain stem
(E) represents a well recognized syndrome involving upper and lower motor neurons and descending autonomic systems

3.19. Horseradish peroxidase (HRP) injected into the sternocleidomastoid muscle would retrogradely label cells in the:
(A) nucleus ambiguus
(B) anterior horns of C1–C5
(C) hypoglossal nucleus
(D) inferior salivatory nucleus
(E) nucleus solitarius

3.20. Injection of horseradish peroxidase (HRP) into the solitary nuclear complex would retrogradely label cells in the:
(A) superior ganglion of cranial nerve IX
(B) hypoglossal nucleus
(C) dorsal root ganglia of C1–C5
(D) inferior ganglion of cranial nerve X
(E) superior ganglion of cranial nerve X

For each numbered item, select the one heading most closely associated with it. Each lettered heading may be selected once, more than once, or not at all.

Questions 3.21–3.24

(A) Lateral lemniscus
(B) Medial lemniscus
(C) Medial longitudinal fasciculus
(D) Inferior cerebellar peduncle
(E) Spinal trigeminal tract

3.21. Descends to the C2 spinal level

3.22. Present in both spinal cord and brain stem beneath ventricle system

3.23. Formed by decussating internal arcuate fibers

3.24. Contains largely crossed fibers that terminate in the caudal mesencephalon

Questions 3.25–3.28

(A) General somatic efferent (GSE)
(B) Special somatic efferent (SSA)
(C) Special visceral afferent (SVA)
(D) Special visceral efferent (SVE)
(E) General somatic afferent (GSA)

3.25. Descend in inferior vestibular nucleus

3.26. Descend in spinal trigeminal tract

3.27. Enter the tractus solitarius

3.28. Partially encircles the abducens nucleus

Questions 3.29–3.32

(A) Substance P
(B) Acetylcholine
(C) Serotonin
(D) Norepinephrine
(E) Enkephalin

3.29. Nucleus raphe magnus

3.30. Lateral reticular formation of medulla and pons

3.31. Hypoglossal nucleus and dorsal motor nucleus of vagus

3.32. Trigeminal ganglion and spinal trigeminal nucleus

For each numbered item, select the letter designating the part in Fig. 3.1 which matches it correctly. A lettered part may be selected once, more than once, or not at all.

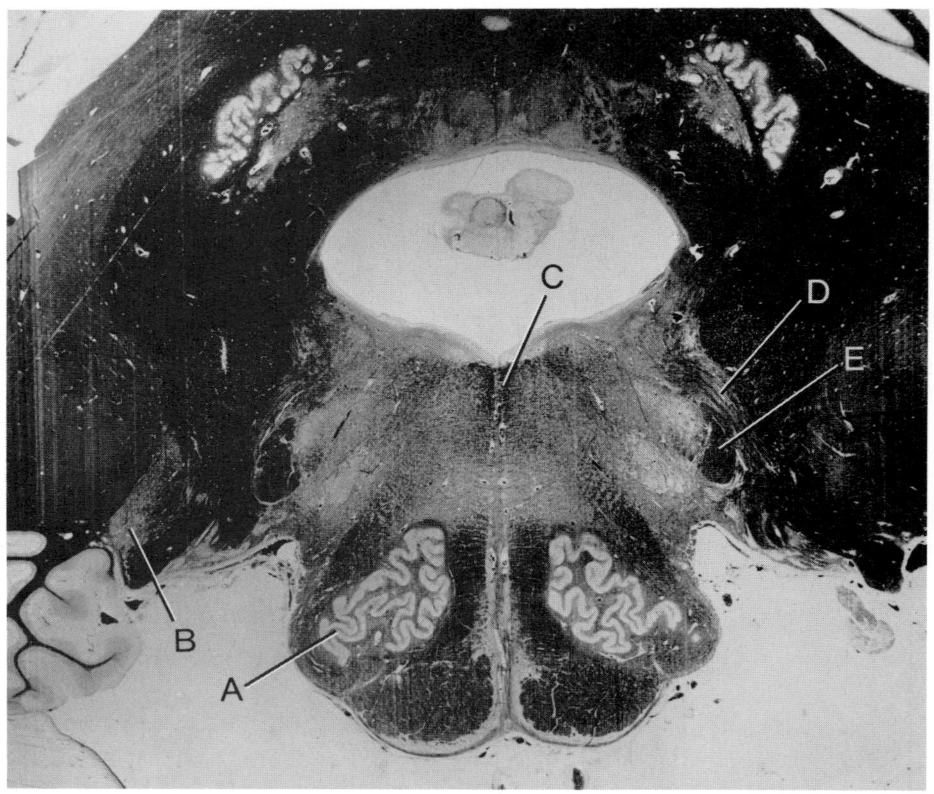

Figure 3.1. Transverse Weigert-stained section of the brain stem through the upper medulla and cerebellum. (From H. A. Riley, *Atlas of the Basal Ganglia, Brain Stem and Spinal Cord*, 1943; courtesy of Williams & Wilkins, Baltimore.)

3.33. Composed of primary general somatic afferent fibers

3.34. Projects fibers to the cerebellar cortex and receives input from the deep cerebellar nuclei

3.35. Projects fibers to parts of all vestibular nuclei

3.36. Afferents arise from the spiral ganglion

For each numbered item, select the letter designating the part in Fig. 3.2 which matches it correctly. A lettered part may be selected once, more than once, or not at all.

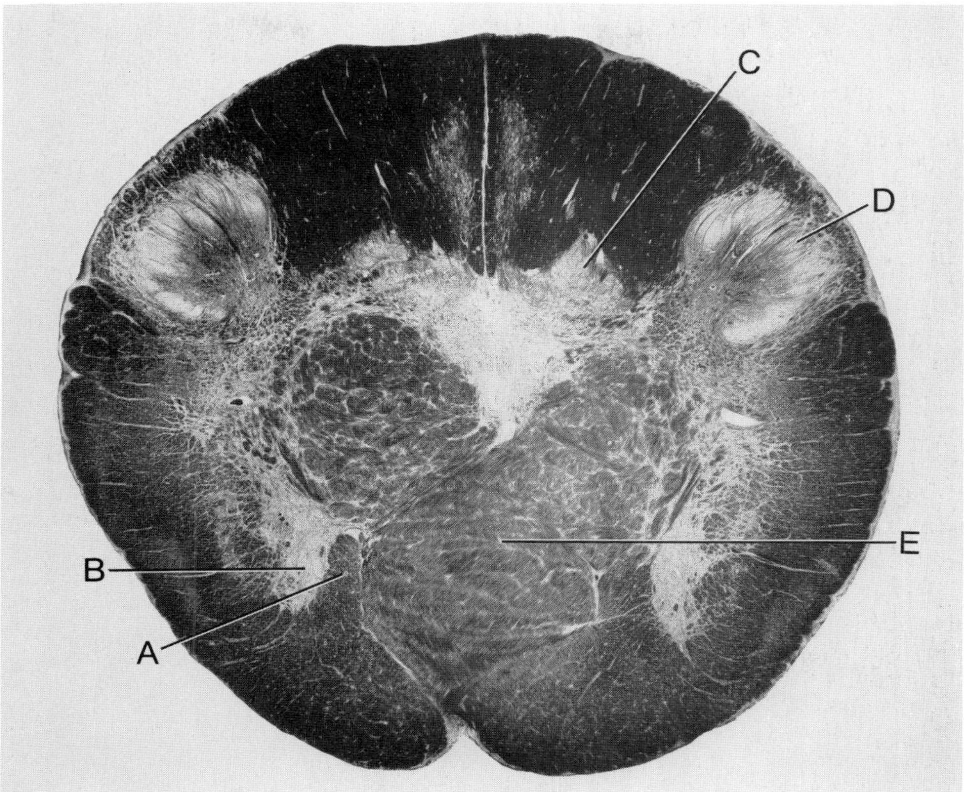

Figure 3.2. Transverse Weigert-stained section through the caudal medulla. (From H. A. Riley, *Atlas of the Basal Ganglia, Brain Stem and Spinal Cord*, 1943; courtesy of Williams & Wilkins, Baltimore.)

3.37. Supraspinal nucleus

3.38. Efferent fibers form part of the medial lemniscus

3.39. Concerned particularly with pain and thermal sense

3.40. A lesion in this region would produce an upper motor neuron paralysis bilaterally

For each numbered item, select the letter designating the part in Fig. 3.3 which matches it correctly. A lettered part may be selected once, more than once, or not at all.

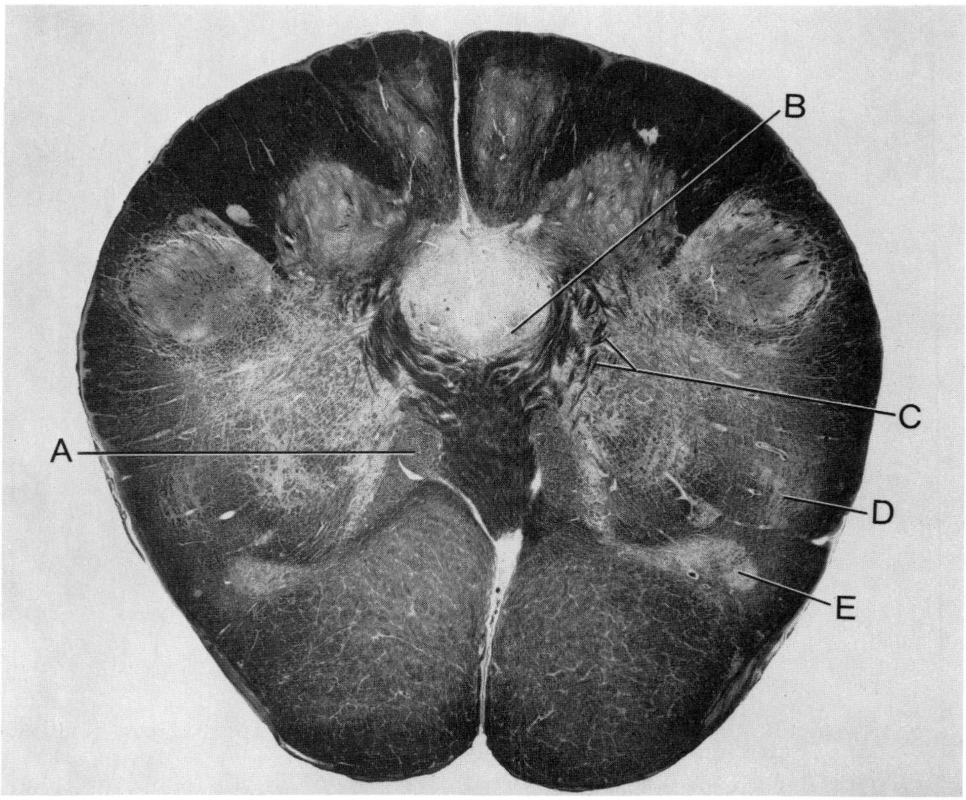

Figure 3.3. Transverse weigert-stained section through the caudal medulla. (From H. A. Riley, *Atlas of the Basal Ganglia, Brain Stem and Spinal Cord*, 1943; courtesy of Williams & Wilkins, Baltimore.)

3.41. Internal arcuate fibers

3.42. General somatic efferent cranial nerve nucleus

3.43. Contains mainly pontine reticulospinal fibers

3.44. Medullary cerebellar relay nucleus which receives collaterals from the spinothalamic tracts

For each numbered item, select the letter designating the part in Fig. 3.4 which matches it correctly. A lettered part may be selected once, more than once, or not at all.

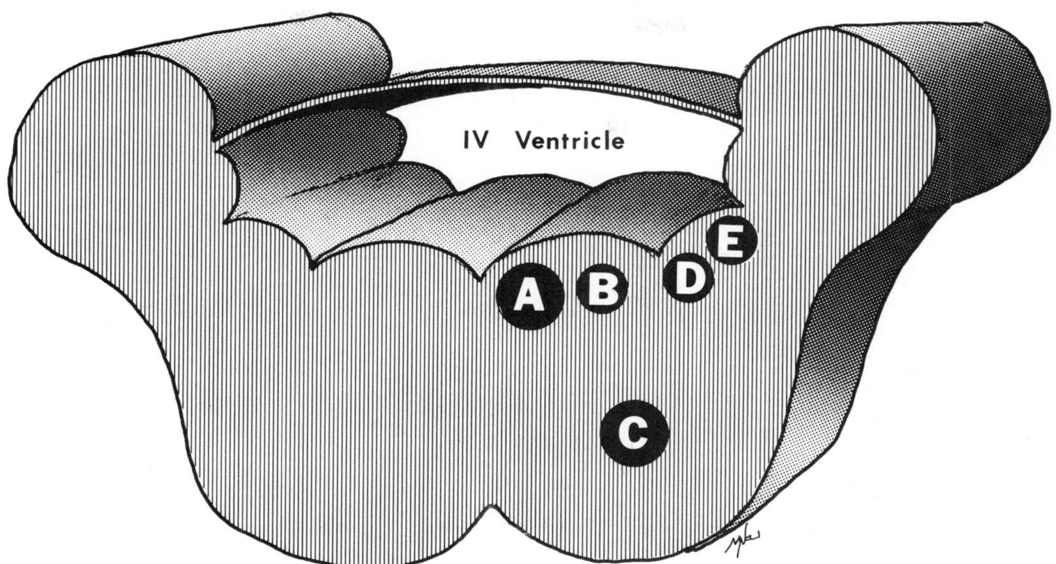

Figure 3.4. Schematic drawing of the caudal brain stem.

3.45. Special visceral efferent (SVE) cell column

3.46. Special visceral afferent (SVA) cell column

3.47. General visceral efferent (GVA) cell column

3.48. General somatic efferent (GSE) cell column

For each numbered item, indicate whether it is associated with

A only (A)
B only (B)
Both A and B (C)
Neither A or B (D)

Questions 3.49–3.52

(A) Solitary nuclear complex
(B) Spinal trigeminal nuclear complex
(C) Both
(D) Neither

3.49. Receives primary afferents from cranial nerves VII, IX, and X

3.50. Projects fibers to phrenic nerve nucleus

3.51. Gives rises to uncrossed ascending sensory pathway

3.52. Projects fibers to cerebellum

Questions 3.53–3.56

(A) Lateral and rostral solitary nuclei
(B) Caudal and medial solitary nuclei
(C) Both
(D) Neither

3.53. General visceral afferents

3.54. Project to parabrachial and thalamic nuclei

3.55. Commissural nucleus of the vagus nerve

3.56. Project to respiratory centers in the rostral pons and cervical spinal cord

For each of the incomplete statements below, *one* or *more* of the completions given is correct. Choose answer:

(A) Only **1, 2,** and **3** are correct
(B) Only **1** and **3** are correct
(C) Only **2** and **4** are correct
(D) Only **4** is correct
(E) **All** are correct

3.57. A complete lesion of the vagus nerve on one side is associated with:
(1) paralysis of pharynx and larynx
(2) hoarseness of the voice
(3) deviation of the uvula to the normal side on phonation
(4) regurgitation of fluids through the nose

3.58. The floor of the fourth ventricle overlies which of the following structures:
(1) hypoglossal nucleus
(2) vestibular nuclei
(3) dorsal motor nucleus of the vagus
(4) area postrema

3.59. The spinal trigeminal tract:
(1) is topographically organized in an inverted fashion
(2) contains only general somatic afferent fibers
(3) contains afferents from cranial nerves VII, IX, and X
(4) is composed of second order neurons

3.60. The nucleus ambiguus:
(1) gives rise to general visceral efferent (GVE) fibers
(2) gives rise to fibers that pass with parts of cranial nerves IX, X, and XI
(3) can be defined only in a physiological sense
(4) innervates the muscles of the larynx and pharynx

3.61. Corticobulbar fibers synapsing directly upon motor cranial nerve nuclei terminate upon:
(1) hypoglossal nucleus
(2) trigeminal motor nucleus
(3) facial nucleus
(4) abducens nucleus

3.62. Inferior alternating hemiplegia involves:
(1) the medullary pyramid and often the medial lemniscus
(2) only the internal arcuate fibers
(3) fibers of the hypoglossal nerve
(4) fibers of the vagus nerve

3.63. The neural pathways in the hiccup reflex involve:
(1) afferent fibers of the vagus nerve
(2) nuclei of the solitary fasciculus
(3) cells of the phrenic nerve nucleus at C3, C4, and C5
(4) the carotid sinus nerve

3.64. A patient with lateral medullary syndrome is likely to exhibit:
(1) ipsilateral facial analgesia
(2) contralateral body hemianesthesia
(3) ataxia
(4) hoarseness of the voice

3.65. Fibers projecting to the cerebellum via the inferior cerebellar peduncle arise from:

(1) nuclei at multiple spinal levels
(2) dorsal root ganglia
(3) medullary relay nuclei
(4) pontine relay nuclei

3.66. The spinal trigeminal nucleus:

(1) is cytologically divisible into three rostrocaudal subdivisions
(2) is topographically organized dorsoventrally
(3) extends from the rostral pons to C2
(4) is laminated like the dorsal horn of the spinal gray

3.67. The special visceral efferent (SVE) cell column in the brain stem includes:

(1) the nucleus ambiguus
(2) neurons forming the spinal part of the accessory nerve
(3) the facial motor nucleus
(4) the hypoglossal nucleus

Questions 3.68–3.71

The numbered outline drawings of spinal cord and medulla in Fig. 3.5 have lesions indicated by *hatched areas*. Use these figures to answer questions 3.68 through 3.71.

(A) Only **1, 2,** and **3** are correct
(B) Only **1** and **3** are correct
(C) Only **2** and **4** are correct
(D) Only **4** is correct
(E) **All** are correct

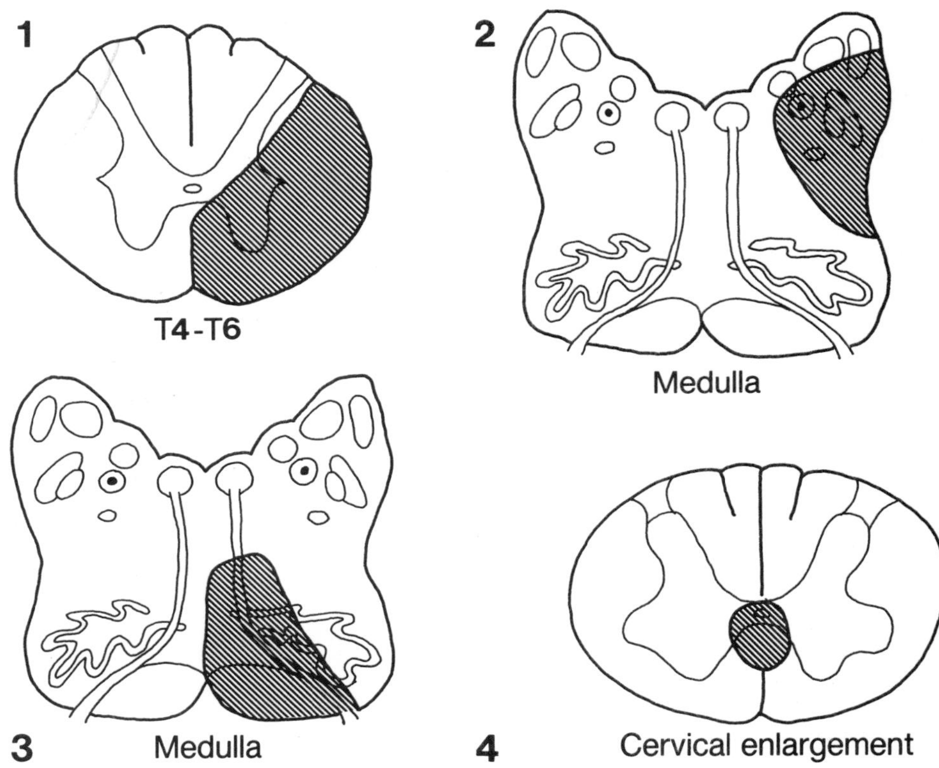

Figure 3.5

3.68. Lesions producing paresis, hyper-reflexia and the Babinski sign

3.69. Lesions associated with paralysis and muscle atrophy

3.70. Associated with bilateral loss of pain and thermal sense

3.71. Neurological deficits correspond only with the level of the lesion

For each of the incomplete statements below, *one* or *more* of the completions given is correct. Choose answer:

(A) Only **1, 2,** and **3** are correct
(B) Only **1** and **3** are correct
(C) Only **2** and **4** are correct
(D) Only **4** is correct
(E) **All** are correct

3.72. Pathways conveying taste sensation involve:
(1) the geniculate and inferior glossopharyngeal and vagal ganglia
(2) lateral and rostral cell columns of the solitary nucleus
(3) ipsilateral secondary brain stem pathways
(4) contralateral specific thalamic relay nuclei

3.73. Aside from the reticular formation, medullary nuclei involved in driving respiration include the:
(1) nucleus ambiguus
(2) dorsal motor nucleus of the vagus
(3) hypoglossal nucleus
(4) solitary nuclear complex

3.74. Cranial nerves giving rise to descending fibers in the brain stem include:
(1) vestibular
(2) trigeminal
(3) vagus and glossopharyngeal
(4) cochlear

3.75. The salivatory nuclear complex
(1) is located at midmedullary levels
(2) is easily recognized in Nissl-stained material
(3) gives rise to SVE fibers
(4) projects fibers to *both* the otic and submandibular ganglia

3.76. Pseudobulbar palsy is associated with:
(1) weakness in muscles associated with chewing, swallowing and breathing
(2) muscle atrophy
(3) emotional instability
(4) detectable sensory loss

3.77. The accessory cuneate nucleus:
(1) receives projections from cervical spinal ganglia
(2) is the medullary equivalent of the dorsal nucleus of Clarke
(3) is somatotopically organized
(4) receives afferent from muscle spindles and Golgi tendon organs

3.78. The inferior olivary complex:
(1) gives rise to climbing fibers in the cerebellar cortex
(2) receives projections from spinal cord, the red nucleus, and the deep cerebellar nuclei
(3) projects only crossed fibers to the cerebellum
(4) receives no afferents from the cerebral cortex

Questions 3.79–3.81

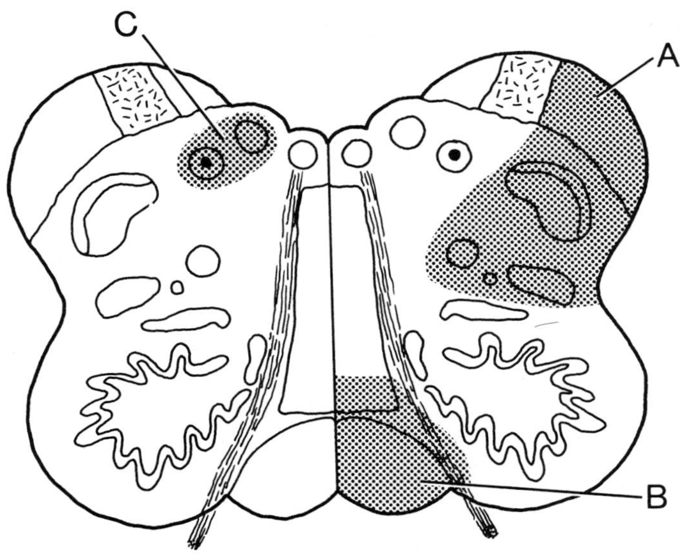

Figure 3.6

3.79. Neurological disturbances resulting from *lesion A* in Fig. 3.6 include:

(1) hoarseness, dysphagia
(2) ipsilateral loss of pain and thermal sense in the face
(3) ipsilateral Horner's syndrome
(4) inability to protrude the tongue

3.80. Neurological disturbances resulting from *lesion B* in Fig. 3.6 include:

(1) ipsilateral paralysis of tongue musculature
(2) some loss of tactile discrimination and kinesthesis in the contralateral upper extremity
(3) contralateral hemiplegia
(4) substantial atrophy of muscles of the contralateral upper extremity

3.81. Neurological disturbances resulting from *lesion C* in Fig. 3.6 would include:

(1) parotid gland dysfunction
(2) loss of carotid sinus reflex
(3) loss of some ipsilateral taste sensation
(4) hoarseness of voice

Answers and Explanations*

3.1. **D**

3.2. **E** See Fig. 5-14, p. 118

3.3. **D** See p. 127

3.4. **A** Pelvic parasympathetic from sacral segments 2, 3, and 4 innervate the detrusor muscle

3.5. **C** Called the lateral medullary syndrome (Wallenberg) due to occlusion of the posterior inferior cerebellar artery or direct branches of the vertebral artery; see pp. 408–409

3.6. **B** With the vocal folds adducted asphyxia is possible unless a tracheostomy is performed; see p. 127

3.7. **A** The object of the procedure is to preserve some tactile sense and the corneal reflex; see p. 108

3.8. **D** Ascending branches of dorsal roots C5, C6, and C7 ascend in the fasciculus cuneatus and terminate upon cells in both the cuneate and accessory cuneate nuclei; see p. 83

3.9. **D** See p. 130

3.10. **B** Increases in carotid arterial pressure excite carotid baroreceptors. Glossopharyngeal afferents to the nucleus solitarius ultimately impinge upon the dorsal motor nucleus of the vagus which bring about reductions in heart rate and arterial blood pressure; see pp. 127–128

3.11. **C** See p. 127

3.12. **B** See pp. 102 and 108

3.13. **E** See pp. 75 and 106

3.14. **B** See p. 119

3.15. **C** See p. 119

3.16. **D** See p. 186

3.17. **E** See pp. 112–113

3.18. **B** See p. 130

3.19. **B** See p. 121

3.20. **D** General and special visceral afferent fibers arise from the inferior vagal ganglion (nodosal ganglion); see p. 121

3.21. **E** See pp. 107–108

3.22. **C** See pp. 94 and 115

3.23. **B** See pp. 75 and 106

3.24. **A** See p. 141

3.25. **B** See p. 119

3.26. **E** See pp. 106–107 and 119

3.27. **C** See pp. 121–125

3.28. **D** See p. 149

3.29. **C** See pp. 113–114 and Figs. 5-11 and 5-12

3.30. **D** See p. 118

3.31. **B** See p. 118

3.32. **A** See p. 119

3.33. **E** Spinal trigeminal tract

3.34. **A** Inferior olivary complex

3.35. **D** Vestibular nerve root

3.36. **B** Ventral cochlear nucleus

3.37. **B**

3.38. **C** Nucleus cuneatus

3.39. **D** Spinal trigeminal nucleus

3.40. **E** Decussation of corticospinal tracts

3.41. **C**

3.42. **B** Hypoglossal nucleus

3.43. **A** Medial longitudinal fasciculus; see p. 115

3.44. **D** Lateral reticular nucleus of medulla

3.45. **C** Represented by the nucleus ambiguus

3.46. **D** Represented by the nucleus solitarius. Part of this cell column also receives general visceral afferents

3.47. **B** Represented by the dorsal motor nucleus of the vagus

* All page numbers and illustration citations refer to Carpenter: CORE TEXT OF NEUROANATOMY, 3rd edition; © 1985, Williams & Wilkins.

3.48. **A** Represented in the medulla by the hypoglossal nucleus

3.49. **C** See p. 108

3.50. **A** See p. 95 and Fig. 4-15

3.51. **A** See p. 125 and Fig. 5-21

3.52. **B** See pp. 109 and 159

3.53. **B** See p. 125

3.54. **C** See p. 125

3.55. **B** See p. 125

3.56. **C** See pp. 95 and 126

3.57. **E** See p. 127

3.58. **A** See pp. 42 and 110; Fig. 5-15

3.59. **B** Composed of fibers of first order neurons, most of which are GSA. Some GVA fibers in the tract project to the solitary nucleus

3.60. **C** This nucleus is well named but can be identified in Nissl preparations; see p. 127

3.61. **A** Direct corticobulbar fibers to these motor cranial nerve nuclei are bilateral and nearly equal, except for those terminating in the ventral part of the facial nucleus; see p. 130

3.62. **B** This is the syndrome associated with occlusion of the anterior spinal artery close to its origin from the vertebral artery; see p. 407 and Fig. 14-1

3.63. **A** Hiccup involves periodic uncontrolled brisk contractions of the diaphragm. Afferent input is via the vagus nerve; see Fig. 4-15 and p. 95

3.64. **E** All of these may be associated with the lateral medullary syndrome (Wallenberg) which appears with variations. Syndrome is associated with occlusion of the posterior inferior cerebellar artery or direct bulbar branches of the vertebral artery; see pp. 407–408

3.65. **B** See p. 115

3.66. **E** See pp. 108–109, 156–157, and Figs. 5-8 and 6-21

3.67. **B** See p. 119; neurons at C1 and C5 which give rise to the spinal part of the accessory nerve are not classified as SVE

3.68. **B** Both lesions involve fibers of the corticospinal tract

3.69. **A** All three of these lesions involve spinal and cranial nerve fibers and would produce lower motor neuron disturbances

3.70. **C** The lesion at *2* would interrupt fibers of the spinal trigeminal and the spinothalamic tracts, producing sensory loss in different locations on both sides of the body. The lesion in *4* would bilaterally interrupt crossing fibers of the spinothalamic tracts

3.71. **D** Only in *4* would the sensory loss correspond fairly closely with the level of the lesion

3.72. **A** Ascending taste pathways are uncrossed; see Fig. 5-21

3.73. **D** Solitary nuclear complex; see pp. 95 and 126; also Fig. 4-15

3.74. **A** The first three give rise to descending fibers in the inferior vestibular nucleus, the spinal trigeminal tract and the solitary tract; see Fig. 5-16

3.75. **D** See pp. 128 and 151 and Fig. 6-18

3.76. **B** See p. 130

3.77. **E** See pp. 83 and 106

3.78. **A** The inferior olivary complex receives afferent fibers from the cerebellar cortex; see p. 111

3.79. **A** The lesion at *A* does not involve the hypoglossal nerve or nucleus

3.80. **B** Contralateral sensory loss would be relatively minor and, if present would involve the lower extremity; ventral parts of the medial lemniscus contain fibers originating in the nucleus gracilis. There would be no atrophy in the contralateral upper extremity

3.81. **A** Lesion involves general and special visceral afferent fibers as well as general visceral efferent fibers of the glossopharyngeal and vagus nerves

4

Pons

Questions

Select the one best answer

4.1. The olivocochlear bundle:
- (A) is concerned with "auditory sharpening"
- (B) consists of both crossed and uncrossed fibers which emerge from the brain stem with the vestibular nerve
- (C) innervates the stapedius muscle
- (D) is associated with the phenomenon of paracusis
- (E) conveys impulses only to specific parts of the cochlea

4.2. Primary auditory fibers are distributed:
- (A) so that fibers from the apex of the cochlear terminate in the dorsal cochlear nucleus
- (B) to all cochlear nuclei and each cochlear nucleus has a full tonotopic spectrum
- (C) to all cochlear nuclei with lower frequencies represented dorsally
- (D) in the cochlear nuclei with higher frequencies represented dorsally in all major divisions
- (E) tonotopically in the two divisions of the ventral cochlear nucleus

4.3. The principal ascending auditory pathway in the brain stem is:
- (A) medial lemniscus
- (B) trapezoid body
- (C) ventral acoustic stria
- (D) lateral lemniscus
- (E) acoustic tubercle

4.4. In the auditory system:
- (A) parts of all relay nuclei from the end organ to the gyrus of Heschl are tonotopically organized
- (B) multiple tonotopic organizations are present in all divisions of the cochlear nuclei, the inferior colliculus, and the medial geniculate body
- (C) ascending fibers in the brain stem, of the second and higher orders, are exclusively crossed
- (D) the lateral lemniscus terminates in the parvicellular part of the medial geniculate body
- (E) the only brain stem decussation of auditory fibers forms the trapezoid body

4.5. Secondary auditory fibers from the dorsal and ventral cochlear nuclei project to, or ascend in, all of the following structures, *except*:
- (A) reticular formation
- (B) superior olivary nucleus
- (C) ipsilateral lateral lemniscus
- (D) nuclei of the trapezoid body
- (E) contralateral lateral lemniscus

4.6. Primary vestibular fibers:
- (A) project upon the vestibular nuclei and specific parts of the cerebellar cortex
- (B) pass to all parts of the vestibular nuclei and to the fastigial nuclei
- (C) ascend in the medial longitudinal fasciculus (MLF) to the nuclei of the extraocular muscles
- (D) project bilaterally to the vestibular nuclei
- (E) project ipsilaterally to the vestibular nuclei and the reticular formation

4.7. Lesions of the spinal trigeminal tract result chiefly in:
(A) loss of pain, thermal, and tactile sense
(B) loss of tactile sense
(C) loss of kinesthetic sense and two-point discrimination
(D) loss of pain and thermal sense
(E) loss of pain

4.8. Trigeminal sensory relay nuclei project impulses to the thalamus:
(A) via the spinothalamic tracts
(B) via the contralateral ventral trigeminothalamic and dorsal trigeminal tracts
(C) via the mesencephalic root
(D) in association with the contralateral medial lemniscus and in the ipsilateral dorsal trigeminal tract
(E) in the ventral trigeminothalamic tract and the brain stem reticular formation

4.9. A voluntary central type facial palsy:
(A) involves only muscles in the lower part of the face ipsilaterally
(B) results in a relatively mild lower facial weakness and loss of the corneal reflex
(C) is due to involvement of crossed corticobulbar fibers
(D) results from a brain stem lesion destroying fibers of the facial nerve
(E) is a consequence of destruction of reticular neurons which project to particular parts of the facial nucleus

4.10. General visceral efferent (GVE) fibers of cranial nerve VII arise in the:
(A) solitary nucleus
(B) superior salivatory nucleus
(C) inferior salivatory nucleus
(D) geniculate ganglion
(E) motor nucleus of VII

4.11. Afferent trigeminal nerve fibers associated with proprioception and stretch receptors have their cell bodies in:
(A) ophthalmic division of trigeminal ganglion
(B) maxillary division of trigeminal ganglion
(C) mesencephalic nucleus of V
(D) mandibular division of trigeminal ganglion
(E) all parts of the trigeminal ganglion

4.12. A brain stem lesion associated with horizontal diplopia on attempted gaze to the right, a left hemiplegia, and impaired kinesthetic and discriminative tactile sense on the left most likely involves:
(A) structures in the cerebellopontine tegmentum
(B) the abducens nucleus and the pontine tegmentum
(C) the basal part of the pons on the right and the adjacent ventral pontine tegmentum
(D) the ventromedial part of the midbrain tegmentum and the crus cerebri on the right
(E) the medullary pyramid and medial lemniscus on the right

4.13. A patient with a peripheral facial palsy, loss of taste in the anterior ⅔ of the tongue, hyperacusis, impaired salivary secretion, and profuse lacrimation in response to a salivary stimulus, has had a:
(A) lesion in the major superficial petrosal nerve or in the pterygopalatine ganglion
(B) lesion distal to the geniculate ganglion
(C) partial lesion of the facial nerve at the stylomastoid foramen
(D) lesion of the geniculate ganglion
(E) complete lesion of the facial and intermediate nerves proximal to the geniculate ganglion

4.14. Hyperacusis associated with Bell's palsy results from:
(A) a lesion of the facial nerve at the stylomastoid foramen
(B) a central type facial palsy
(C) paralysis of the tensor tympani muscle
(D) paralysis of the stapedius muscle
(E) inefficient impedence matching in the ossicular chain

4.15. In right lateral gaze paralysis and the syndrome of the medial longitudinal fasciculus (right side) there are common features:
(A) paresis of ocular adduction on attempted gaze to the side of the lesion
(B) monocular horizontal nystagmus
(C) ascending degeneration in the ipsilateral medial longitudinal fasciculus (MLF)
(D) paresis of ocular adduction on attempted gaze to the side opposite the lesion
(E) paresis of ocular adduction on attempted lateral gaze, but this paresis occurs on opposite sides

4.16. If stimulation of the cornea with a wisp of cotton produces only contralateral blinking and closure of the eye, the patient has:

(A) a lesion involving secondary trigeminal fibers
(B) a central type facial palsy
(C) an injury to the ophthalmic division of nerve V
(D) an ipsilateral peripheral facial palsy
(E) impaired corneal sensation ipsilaterally

4.17. In lateral gaze paralysis:

(A) the eyes are forcefully deviated to the side of the lesion
(B) ocular disturbances are due solely to lower motor neuron involvement
(C) the lesion involves cells of the abducens nucleus and internuclear neurons
(D) the lesion involves the medial longitudinal fasciculus
(E) the lesion involves the abducens nerve and adjacent parts of the reticular formation

4.18. Secondary trigeminal afferents are involved in all of the following reflexes, *except*:

(A) corneal
(B) lacrimal
(C) sneezing
(D) mesenteric (jaw jerk)
(E) vomiting

4.19. Branches of the trigeminal nerve convey tactile, thermal, and pain sensation for all of the following, *except*:

(A) mucous membranes of the nasal sinuses
(B) oral cavity
(C) teeth
(D) cutaneous regions of the face and scalp
(E) dura of the posterior fossa

4.20. A lesion in right medial longitudinal fasciculus (MLF) rostral to the abducens nucleus produces:

(A) paralysis of right lateral gaze
(B) horizontal diplopia on the right gaze
(C) impairment of ocular convergence
(D) paralysis of ocular adduction on attempted lateral gaze to the left
(E) monocular horizontal nystagmus on attempted lateral gaze to the right

For each numbered item, select the one heading most closely associated with it. Each lettered heading may be selected once, more than once, or not at all.

Questions 4.21–4.24

(A) Trigeminal ganglion
(B) Principal sensory nucleus of V
(C) Spinal trigeminal nucleus
(D) Mesencephalic nucleus of V
(E) Motor nucleus of V

4.21. Uniquely concerned with pain and thermal sense

4.22. Controls the force of the bite

4.23. Conveys impulses from stretch receptors

4.24. Receives collaterals from primary sensory neurons within the central nervous system

Questions 4.25–4.28

(A) Corneal reflex
(B) Hiccup reflex
(C) Tearing reflex
(D) Carotid sinus reflex
(E) Hyperacusis

4.25. Salivatory nucleus and pterygopalatine ganglion

4.26. Phrenic nerve nuclei

4.27. Vagal visceral efferents

4.28. Effected bilaterally by facial nerve fibers

For each numbered item, select the letter designating the part in Fig. 4.1 which matches it correctly. A lettered part may be selected once, more than once, or not at all.

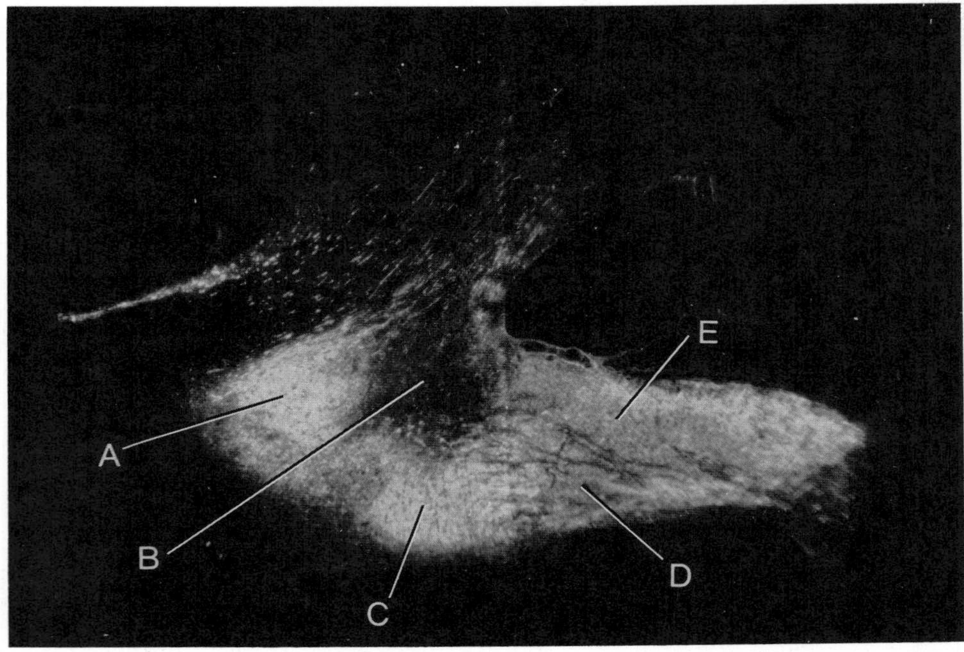

Figure 4.1. Photomicrograph of sagittal autoradiograph through the vestibular nuclei in a monkey. (From M. B. Carpenter and J. Sutin, *Human Neuroanatomy*, 1983; courtesy of Williams and Wilkins, Baltimore.)

4.29. Projects ascending fibers to the ipsilateral trochlear and oculomotor nuclei

4.30. Projects fibers bilaterally and asymmetrically to all nuclei of the extraocular muscles

4.31. Giant cells somatotopically project fibers to lumbosacral spinal segments

4.32. Descending fibers exert facilitating influences upon extensor muscle tone in the ipsilateral upper extremity

For each numbered item, select the one heading most closely associated with it. Each lettered heading may be selected once, more than once, or not at all.

Questions 4.33–4.36

(A) Syndrome of "crocodile" tears
(B) Hyperacusis
(C) Corneal reflex
(D) Flattening of the nasolabial fold
(E) Paracusis

4.33. Occurs in all peripheral and voluntary facial palsies

4.34. Due to paralysis of the stapedius muscle

4.35. Not abolished in central type facial palsies

4.36. Produced by aberrant regeneration of preganglionic parasympathetic fibers

For each numbered item, select the letter designating the part in Fig. 4.2 which matches it correctly. A lettered part may be selected once, more than once, or not at all.

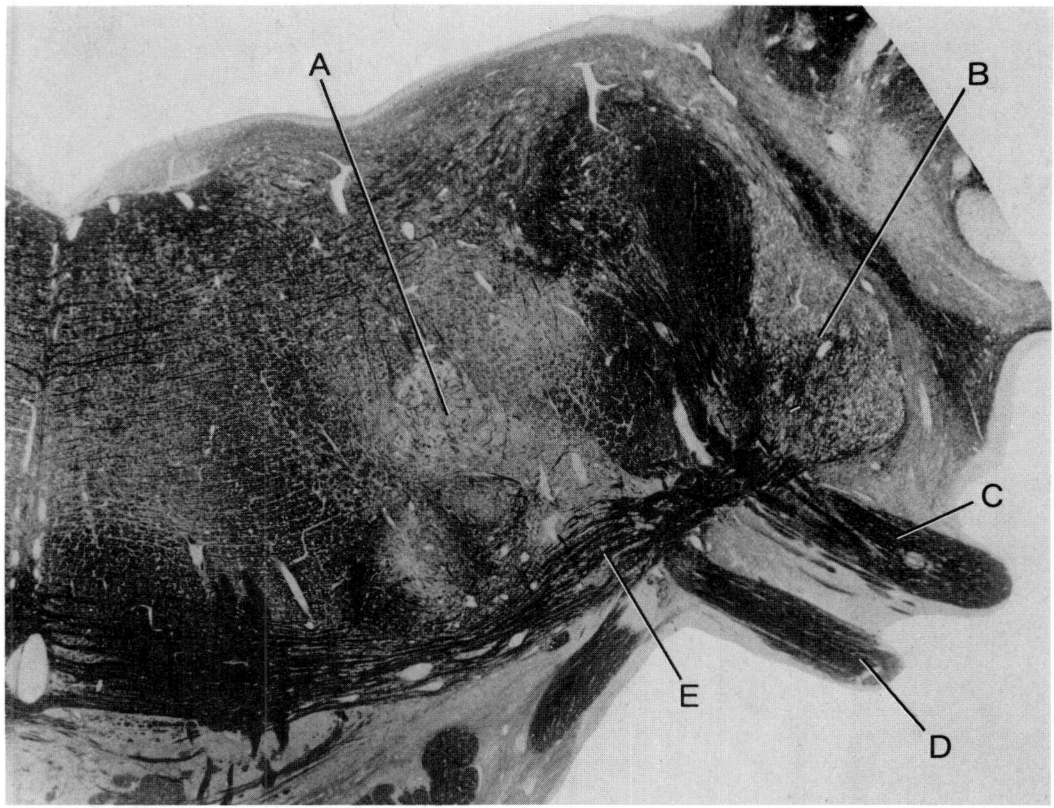

Figure 4.2. Transverse Weigert-stained section through the brain stem at the cerebellopontine angle. (From M. B. Carpenter and J. Sutin, *Human Neuroanatomy*, 1983; courtesy of Williams & Wilkins.)

4.37. Special somatic afferent cranial nerve

4.38. Innervates the buccinator, stapedius, and posterior digastric muscles

4.39. Fibers form the largest auditory decussation

4.40. Nucleus receives special somatic afferent fibers

For each numbered item, select the letter designating the part in Fig. 4.3 which matches it correctly. A lettered part may be selected once, more than once, or not at all.

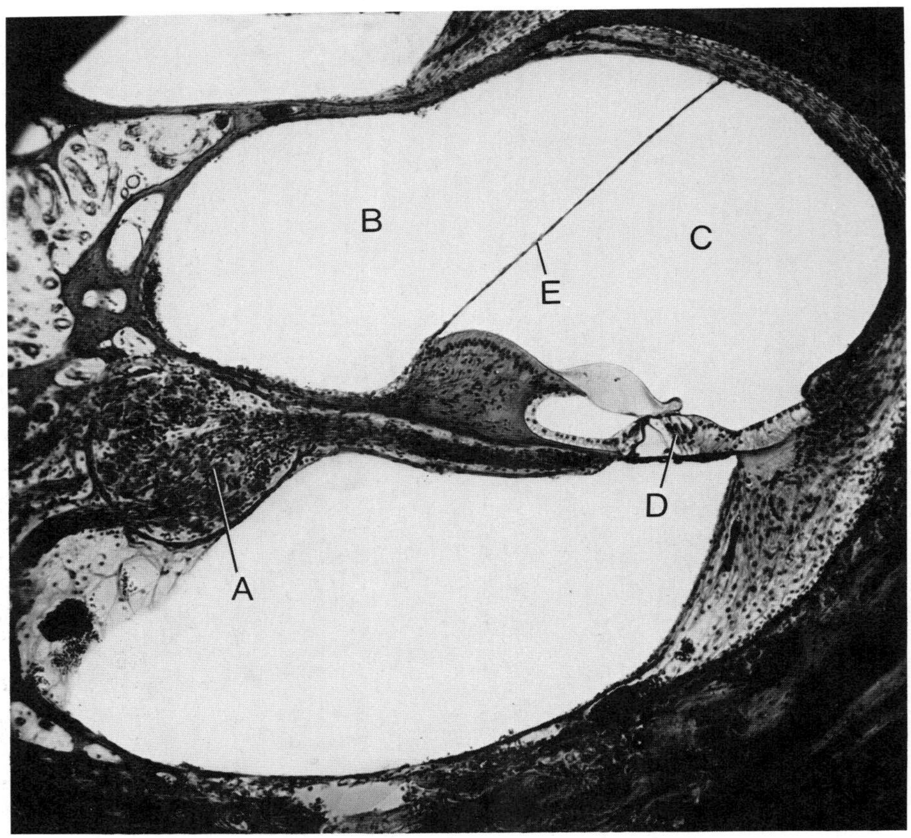

Figure 4.3. Photomicrograph of a radial section through the human cochlea. (From M. B. Carpenter and J. Sutin, *Human Neuroanatomy*, 1983; courtesy of Williams & Wilkins.)

4.41. Receptor cells

4.42. Contains endolymph

4.43. Contains perilymph

4.44. Primary sensory neurons

For each numbered item, select the letter designating the part in Fig. 4.4 which matches it correctly. A lettered part may be selected once, more than once, or not at all.

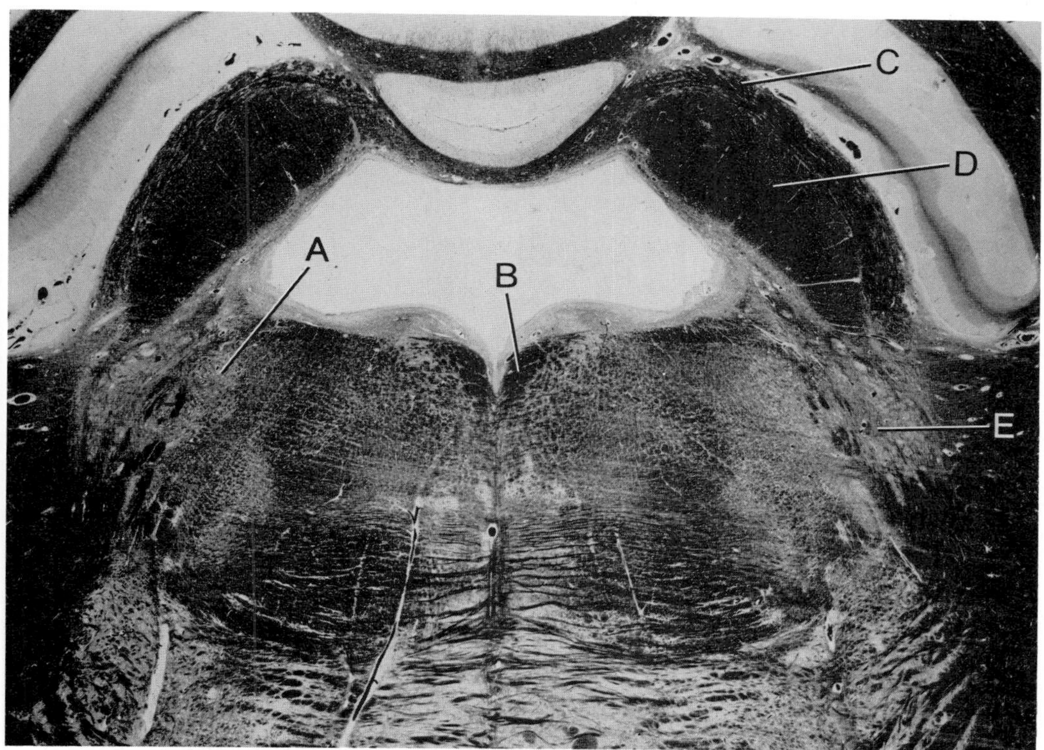

Figure 4.4. Transverse Weigert-stained section through dorsal portions of the rostral pons. (From H. A. Riley, *Atlas of the Basal Ganglia, Brain Stem and Spinal Cord*, 1943; courtesy of Williams & Wilkins, Baltimore.)

4.45. Crossed fibers in this tract originate at spinal levels and project to the cerebellar vermis

4.46. Cells innervate the muscles of mastication

4.47. Ascending fibers in this bundle project to the trochlear and oculomotor nuclei

4.48. Cells in this nucleus receive inputs related to discriminating tactile and pressure sense

For each numbered item, select the letter designating the part in Fig. 4.5 which matches it correctly. A lettered part may be selected once, more than once, or not at all.

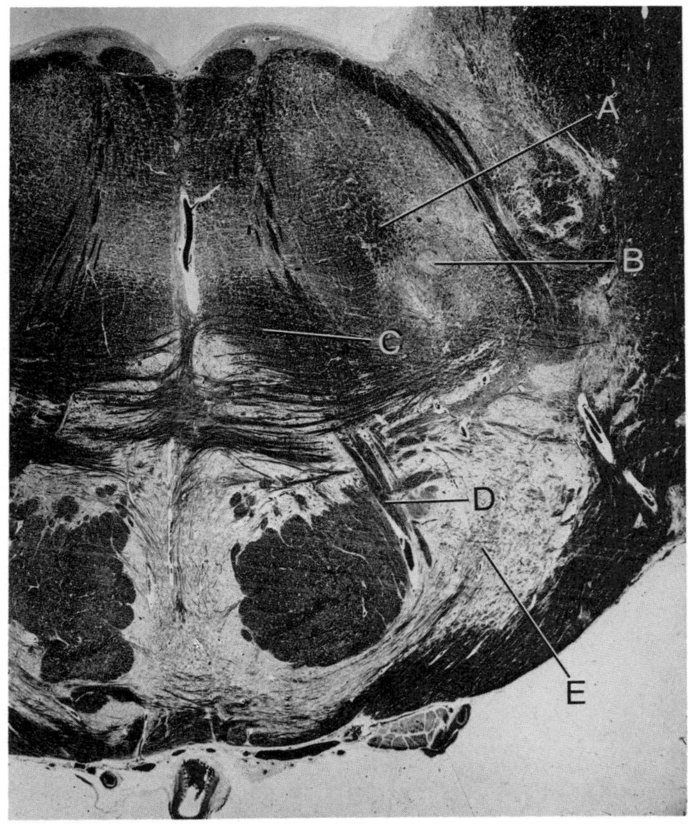

Figure 4.5. Transverse Weigert-stained section through the caudal pons. (From H. A. Riley, *Atlas of the Basal Ganglia, Brain Stem and Spinal Cord*, 1943; courtesy of Williams & Wilkins, Baltimore.)

4.49. General somatic efferent (GSE) cranial nerve

4.50. Involved in electroencephalographic and behavioral arousal

4.51. Special visceral efferent (SVE) cranial nerve nucleus

4.52. Contributes no fibers or collaterals to reticular formation

For each numbered item, select the letter designating the part in Fig. 4.6 which matches it correctly. A lettered part may be selected once, more than once, or not at all.

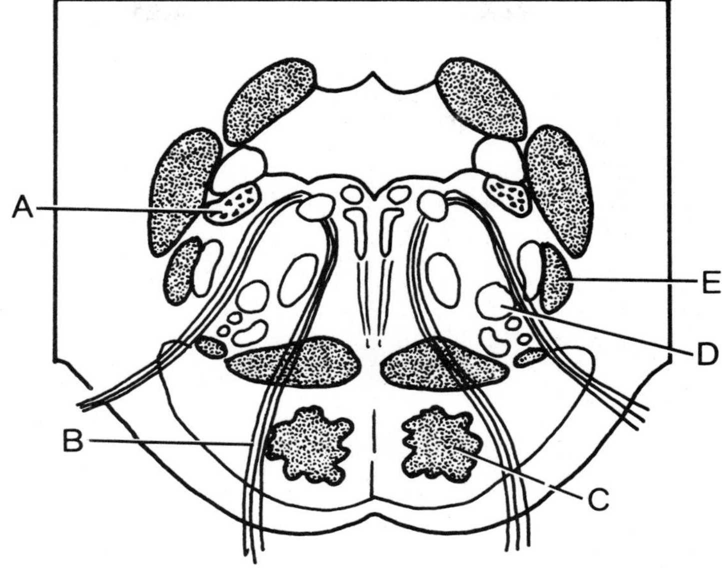

Figure 4.6

4.53. A lesion here would produce paralysis of the facial muscles

4.54. A lesion here would produce a diminution of extensor tonus in the ipsilateral extremities

4.55. A lesion here would produce a loss of pain and temperature sensation in the ipsilateral half of the face

4.56 A lesion here would produce horizontal diplopia

For each numbered item, indicate whether it is associated with

A only (A)
B only (B)
Both A and B (C)
Neither A or B (D)

Questions 4.57–4.60

(A) Abducens motor neurons
(B) Abducens internuclear neurons
(C) Both
(D) Neither

4.57. Horizontal diplopia on lateral gaze to the side of the lesion

4.58. Projects fibers via the medial longitudinal fasciculus (MLF) to the contralateral oculomotor nucleus

4.59. Involved in lateral gaze paralysis

4.60. Receive afferents from the vestibular nuclei

Questions 4.61–4.64

(A) Utricle
(B) Saccule
(C) Both
(D) Neither

4.61. Stimulated by linear acceleration

4.62. Projects afferents upon parts of the lateral and inferior vestibular nuclei

4.63. Association with motion sickness

4.64. Responds to angular accelerations

Questions 4.65–4.68

(A) Vestibular efferent fibers
(B) Cochlear efferent fibers
(C) Both
(D) Neither

4.65. Contain both crossed and uncrossed fibers

4.66. Exert inhibitory effects upon the end organ

4.67. Exert facilitating influences upon all parts of the end organ

4.68. Emerge from the brain stem with the cochlear nerve

For each numbered item, indicate whether it is associated with part *A* or *B* of Fig. 4.7.

A only (A)
B only (B)
Both A and B (C)
Neither A nor B (D)

Questions 4.69–4.72

4.69. Isotope transported via a general somatic efferent cranial nerve

4.70. Terminals labeled in parts of a general somatic efferent cranial nerve nucleus

4.71. Contains lower motor and internuclear neurons, both labeled with isotope

4.72. Isotope surrounds neurons innervating the ipsilateral medial rectus muscle

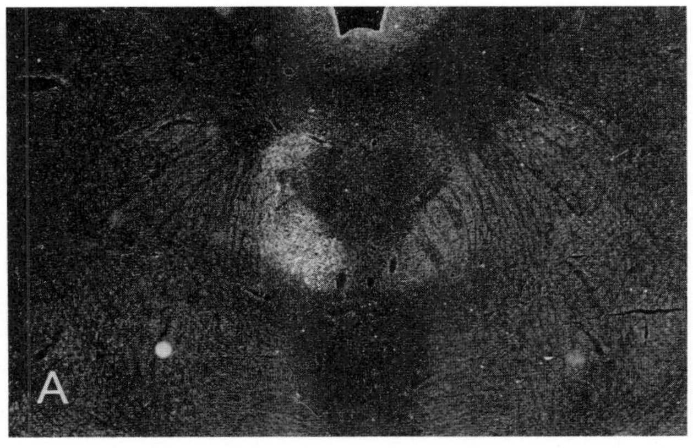

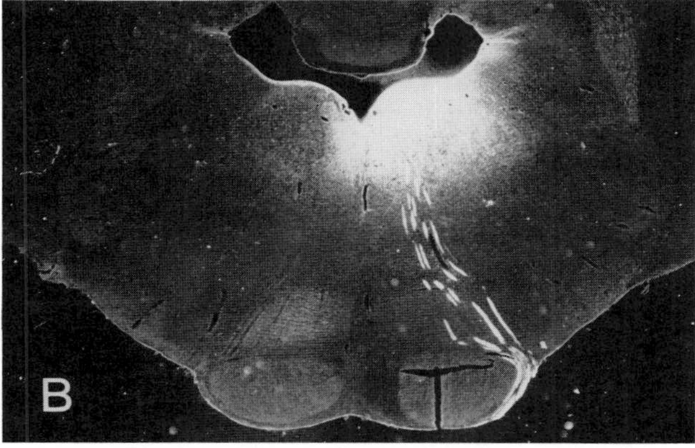

Figure 4.7. Autoradiographs of the brain stem in the monkey: *A*, midbrain; *B*, caudal pons.

For each of the incomplete statements below, *one* or *more* of the completions given is correct. Choose answer:

(A) Only **1, 2,** and **3** are correct
(B) Only **1** and **3** are correct
(C) Only **2** and **4** are correct
(D) Only **4** is correct
(E) **All** are correct

4.73. Primary vestibular afferents related to the macula of the utricle:
(1) arise from cells in the superior vestibular ganglion
(2) arise from cells in the inferior vestibular ganglion
(3) project to the lateral (ventral half) and inferior vestibular nuclei
(4) project to the superior and medial vestibular nuclei

4.74. Corticobulbar fibers:
(1) project bilaterally and directly only to branchiomeric motor cranial nerve nuclei
(2) exert both inhibitory and facilitatory influences upon medullary secondary sensory relay nuclei
(3) destroyed unilaterally result in a mimetic facial palsy
(4) destroyed rostral to the pons result in a contralateral voluntary central type facial palsy

4.75. Descending auditory pathways in the brain stem:
(1) parallel ascending systems
(2) exert inhibitory and facilitatory influences at various levels
(3) play a role in auditory sharpening
(4) are known as the efferent cochlear bundle

4.76. The auditory nerve:
(1) represents the central processes of bipolar cells of the spiral ganglion
(2) gives rise to the acoustic striae which partially decussate
(3) projects tonotopically upon all three divisions of the cochlear nuclei
(4) enters the brain stem between the inferior cerebellar peduncle and the spinal trigeminal tract

4.77. The abducens nucleus:
(1) lies under the facial colliculus
(2) projects to part of the contralateral oculomotor complex
(3) receives fibers from the vestibular nuclei
(4) innervates the medial rectus muscle

4.78. The facial motor nucleus:
(1) lies dorsomedial to the abducens nucleus
(2) gives rise to general visceral efferent fibers
(3) lies ventral to the superior olive
(4) innervates the stylohyoid and posterior belly of the digastric muscles

4.79. Fiber in the facial nerve, or passing with it in part of its course, include:
(1) special visceral afferents (SVA)
(2) special visceral efferents (SVE)
(3) general visceral efferents (GVE)
(4) general somatic efferents (GSE)

4.80. Postganglionic general visceral efferent fibers of intermediate nerve arise from:
(1) otic ganglion
(2) pterygopalative ganglion
(3) geniculate ganglion
(4) submandibular ganglion

4.81. The abducens nucleus is unique among all cranial nerves because:
(1) it contains two distinct populations of neurons
(2) some cells within this nucleus project to the contralateral oculomotor complex
(3) lesions in the nucleus produce different disturbances than lesions in the root fibers
(4) it receives inputs from the medial vestibular nuclei and the reticular formation

4.82. The efferent cochlear bundle:
(1) consists of only crossed fibers
(2) emerges from the brain stem with the vestibular nerve
(3) exert facilitatory influences upon the outer hair cells
(4) contains fibers which established synaptic contact with outer hair cells and cells of the spiral ganglion

4.83. Caloric testing of the labyrinth by injection of cold water into the external auditory meatus:
(1) sets up convection currents in the endolymphatic fluid
(2) has its most potent influence upon the lateral semicircular duct
(3) produces nystagmus (slow phase) which is correlated with the direction of movement of endolymphatic fluid
(4) rarely causes deviation of the eyes

4.84. Orientation in three-dimensional space is dependent upon input via:
(1) the visual system
(2) the posterior column-medial lemniscal system
(3) the labyrinth
(4) the muscle spindles and Golgi tendon organs

4.85. Primary afferents from the cristae of the semicircular canals:
(1) convey information regarding linear acceleration
(2) convey information regarding angular acceleration
(3) terminate primarily in the lateral vestibular nuclei
(4) terminate mainly in the superior and medial vestibular nuclei

4.86. Axons from the ventral cochlear nucleus may synapse in parts of the:
(1) ipsilateral superior olive
(2) contralateral superior olive
(3) trapezoid nuclei
(4) contralateral inferior colliculus

4.87. Following rotation of patient in a Bárány chair, the following can be correlated with the direction of post-rotatory flow of endolymphatic fluid:
(1) slow phase of nystagmus
(2) postural deviation
(3) deviation of eyes
(4) subjective vertigo

4.88. Primary sensory neurons are found in:
(1) the trigeminal (Gasserian, semilunar) ganglion
(2) the principal trigeminal nucleus
(3) the mesencephalic nucleus of the trigeminal nerve
(4) the spinal trigeminal nucleus

4.89. Cells in and around the superior olivary nuclei:
(1) project fibers to the facial motor nucleus which are involved in reflex functions of the stapedius muscle
(2) can inhibit transmission of auditory impulses at the level of the cochlear nuclei
(3) project rostrally in the lateral lemniscus
(4) can inhibit auditory transmission at the organ of Corti

4.90. The abducens nerve:
(1) is the most frequently injured cranial nerve
(2) traverses the cavernous sinus close to the carotid artery
(3) nucleus constitutes an integrative site for horizontal gaze
(4) when injured alone, has no neurological localizing features

For each of the incomplete statements below, *one* or *more* of the completions given is correct. Choose answer:

(A) Only **1, 2,** and **3** are correct
(B) Only **1** and **3** are correct
(C) Only **2** and **4** are correct
(D) Only **4** is correct
(E) **All** are correct

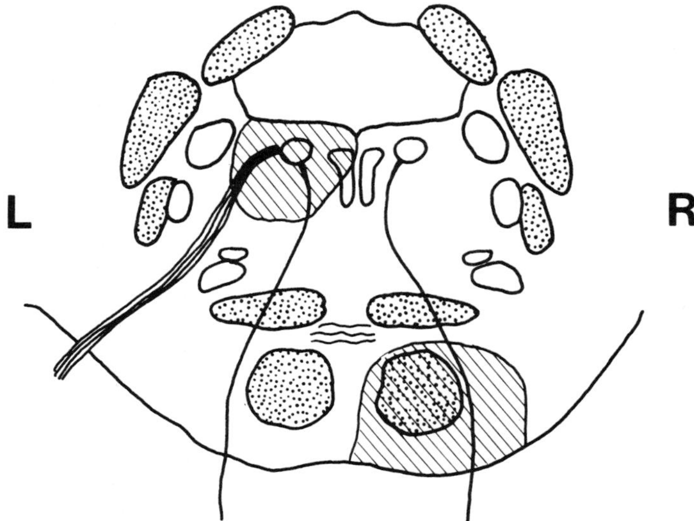

Figure 4.8. Schematic diagram of the caudal pons with lesion areas on the left (*L*) and right (*R*) indicated by *cross-hatching.*

4.91. A lesion encompassing the hatched area on the *right* in Fig. 4.8 might produce:

(1) a middle alternating hemiplegia
(2) ipsilateral horizontal diplopia
(3) a contralateral paralysis of the extremities
(4) contralateral loss of kinesthesis and discriminative tactile sensation

4.92. A lesion encompassing the *hatched area* on the *left* in Fig. 4.8 might produce:

(1) horizontal diplopia
(2) lateral gaze paralysis
(3) paralysis of the contralateral facial muscles
(4) paralysis of the ipsilateral facial muscles

Answers and Explanations*

4.1. **B** Fibers of the olivocochlear bundle are crossed and uncrossed and make synaptic contact with hair cells of the organ of Corti and cells of the spiral ganglion; see p. 141 and Fig. 6-11

4.2. **D** In the cochlear nuclei there is a multiple tonotopic representation with higher frequencies represented dorsally in all divisions; see p. 139

4.3. **D** See p. 141

4.4. **A** In the medial geniculate body only the ventral laminated part is tonotopically organized

4.5. **C** See p. 141

4.6. **A** See pp. 144–145

4.7. **D** Fibers concerned with tactile sense also project to the principal trigeminal nucleus; see p. 157 and Fig. 6-24

4.8. **D** See p. 159 and Fig. 6-23

4.9. **C** See p. 152

4.10. **B** These fibers arise from cells called the superior salivatory cells which are at levels rostral to those of the inferior salivatory nucleus

4.11. **C** These are primary sensory neurons retained within the central nervous system; see p. 158

4.12. **C** Middle alternating hemiplegia in which the lesion involves the corticospinal tract, part of the medial lemniscus, and the root fibers of the cranial nerve VI; see p. 155. Lesion is caused by occlusion of paramedian and short circumferential branches of vertebral artery; see p. 409

4.13. **E** This syndrome results from a lesion proximal to the geniculate ganglia and involves the facial and intermediate nerves. Aberrant regeneration of preganglionic parasympathetic fibers produces the syndrome of "crocodile tears"; see pp. 151–152 and Fig. 6-18

4.14. **D** Paralysis of the stapedius muscle causes sounds to be abnormally loud because of the loss of dampening which this muscle provides; see p. 151.

4.15. **E** Paresis of ocular adduction in lateral gaze paralysis is to the side of lesion; with a lesion in the right MLF, paresis of ipsilateral ocular adduction is evident on attempted lateral gaze to the opposite side, the left; see Fig. 6-16

4.16. **D** In a peripheral facial palsy, corneal sensation is intact but the ipsilateral corneal reflex is abolished. However, stimulation of the cornea on the lesion side will produce a consensual (contralateral) response

4.17. **C** Lateral gaze paralysis due to a lesion in the abducens nucleus, involves both abducens motor neurons whose fibers emerge via the nerve root and abducens internuclear neurons whose fibers ascend in the opposite MLF. See p. 155

4.18. **D** Afferents from stretch receptors in the muscles of mastication pass via the mesencephalic nucleus of V to the motor nucleus of V; this is a monosynaptic myotatic reflex

4.19. **E** The dura of the posterior fossa is innervated by branches of the vagus and upper cervical spinal nerves; see p. 2

4.20. **D** There is a dissociation of horizontal gaze to the opposite side due to a paralysis of ocular adduct on the right. Syndrome of anterior internuclear ophthalmoplegia; see Fig. 6-16

4.21. **C** See p. 157

4.22. **D** See p. 158

* All page numbers and illustration citations refer to Carpenter: CORE TEXT OF NEUROANATOMY, 3rd edition; © 1985, Williams & Wilkins.

4.23. **D** See p. 158
4.24. **E** The mesencephalic nucleus of V provides collaterals to the motor nucleus of V, which form the reflex arc for a myotatic reflex, the so-called "jaw jerk"
4.25. **C** See p. 151
4.26. **B** Impulses transmitted via the phrenic nerve cause the periodic contracts which cause hiccup
4.27. **D** Vagal visceral efferent fibers cause reductions in heart rate and blood pressure
4.28. **A** Afferent impulses conveyed by trigeminal nerve on one side produce bilateral corneal reflexes, via second order trigeminal connections
4.29. **A** Superior vestibular nucleus
4.30. **E** Medial vestibular nucleus
4.31. **B** Dorsal part of lateral vestibular nucleus; see p. 91
4.32. **C** Ventral part of lateral vestibular nucleus; see Fig. 6-13
4.33. **D** Both peripheral and voluntary facial palsies effect lower facial muscles
4.34. **B** See p. 151
4.35. **C** Reflex arc remains intact
4.36. **A** See p. 152
4.37. **C** Vestibular nerve; see Fig. 6-5
4.38. **D** Facial nerve; see Fig. 6-5
4.39. **E** Ventral acoustic stria
4.40. **B** Ventral cochlear nucleus
4.41. **D** Outer hair cells, organ of Corti
4.42. **C** Cochlear duct
4.43. **B** Scala vestibuli
4.44. **A** Spiral ganglion
4.45. **C** Anterior spinocerebellar tract
4.46. **A** Motor trigeminal nucleus
4.47. **B** Medial longitudinal fasciculus (MLF)
4.48. **E** Principal trigeminal sensory nucleus
4.49. **D** Abducens nerve
4.50. **A** Central tegmental tract
4.51. **B** Facial nucleus
4.52. **C** Medial lemniscus
4.53. **D** Facial nucleus
4.54. **A** Lateral vestibular nucleus
4.55. **E** Spinal trigeminal tract
4.56. **B** Abducens nerve; lesion would produce horizontal diplopia on attempted lateral gaze to that side
4.57. **A** Lesion involving abducens nerve
4.58. **B**
4.59. **C** See p. 155
4.60. **C** See p. 154
4.61. **C** Utricle is stimulated by linear acceleration in the longitudinal axis of the body (e.g., elevator); the saccule is stimulated by linear acceleration in the frontal (anteroposterior) axis of the body. See p. 143
4.62. **A** See p. 144
4.63. **A** The utricle is particularly concerned with motion sickness
4.64. **D** The semicircular ducts respond to angular acceleration
4.65. **C** See pp. 141–142 and 147
4.66. **B** See pp. 141–142
4.67. **A** See p. 147
4.68. **D** Both groups of efferent fibers emerge from the brain stem with the vestibular nerve
4.69. **B** Abducens nerve
4.70. **C** Terminals are labeled in parts of both the abducens and oculomotor nuclei
4.71. **B** Abducens nucleus
4.72. **A** Cells of the medial rectus neurons in the oculomotor nucleus are surrounded by terminals of fibers originating from abducens internuclear neurons in part *B*
4.73. **B** See Fig. 6-12
4.74. **C** See pp. 128–130 and 152–153
4.75. **A** See p. 142
4.76. **B** See pp. 137–139
4.77. **A**
4.78. **D** See p. 151
4.79. **A** See p. 149–151
4.80. **C** The geniculate ganglion is sensory and contains no synapses
4.81. **E** See p. 153
4.82. **C** See pp. 141–142
4.83. **A** See p. 148
4.84. **A** Stretch receptors project most of their impulses to the cerebellum and are not consciously perceived
4.85. **C** See pp. 144–145
4.86. **E** All of these locations

4.87. **A** The subjective sense of vertigo is opposite the direction of rotation

4.88. **B** See pp. 155 and 158

4.89. **E** See p. 142

4.90. **E** See pp. 153–154

4.91. **A** Lesion involves part of the basilar pons, the corticospinal tract, and fibers of the abducens nerve

4.92. **C** Lesion involves the abducens nucleus and the genu of the facial nerve

5

Mesencephalon

Questions

Select the one best answer

. The pupillary light reflex is both direct l consensual because:
(A) retinal axons cross in the optic chiasm
(B) pretectal neurons receive crossed retinal fibers
(C) visceral neurons in the oculomotor complex receive bilateral input from pretectal nuclei
(D) pretectal neurons project bilaterally to the ciliary ganglia
(E) the Edinger-Westphal nucleus projects bilaterally to the ciliary ganglia

5.2. The pretectal nucleus most involved in the pupillary light reflex is:
(A) nucleus of the optic tract
(B) nuclei of posterior commissure
(C) pretectal olivary nucleus
(D) nucleus of the pretectal area
(E) interstitial nucleus of Cajal

5.3. The mesencephalic nucleus of the trigeminal nerve:
(A) receives fibers from the trigeminal ganglion
(B) gives rise to uncrossed ascending fibers in the dorsal trigeminal tract
(C) conveys impulses from stretch receptors in the muscles of mastication, kinesthetic sense and pressure sense
(D) gives rise to fibers that pass exclusively with the third division of cranial nerve V
(E) is formed of cells intermingled at all levels with those of the locus ceruleus

5.4. A complete lesion of the oculomotor nerve results in:
(A) ptosis of the eyelid, an internal strabismus, and severe limitations of ipsilateral eye movements
(B) a fully dilated pupil not responsive to light, but reactive to accommodation
(C) a fully dilated pupil and only a consensual pupillary response to light
(D) a contralateral ptosis and an immobile abducted eye
(E) anisocoria (unequal pupils) with reduction of both direct and consensual pupillary responses to light

5.5. Decerebrate rigidity resulting from intercollicular transection of the brain stem:
(A) is a consequence of bilateral interruption of corticospinal fibers
(B) represents the removal of cortical and diencephalic influences that inhibit brain stem reticular neurons
(C) represents an imbalance of facilitating and inhibiting mechanisms expressed by great overactivity of gamma (γ) motor neurons
(D) is due to overactivity of neurons in the medullary reticular formation
(E) is the consequence of cerebellar influences acting upon the brain stem reticular formation

5.6. A patient with a lesion of the trochlear nerve might have difficulty:
(A) looking upward and outward
(B) crossing his eyes
(C) making conjugate lateral eye movements
(D) walking down stairs
(E) accommodating for near vision

5.7. A large midbrain lesion involving a ventromedial tegmentum and crus cerebri on the right would produce:
(A) decerebrate rigidity on the right
(B) a complete right oculomotor palsy and an incomplete left hemiparesis
(C) unconsciousness, irregular respiration and rapid eye movements
(D) neocerebellar disturbances on the right side
(E) tremor, ataxia, and dysmetria on the right and a complete right oculomotor palsy

5.8. The superior colliculi:
(A) receive afferent fibers from the retinae, the striate (i.e., visual) cortex and the spinal cord
(B) receive crossed fibers from the optic tract, uncrossed fibers from the striate cortex, and project bilaterally to the oculomotor complex
(C) are concerned with vertical and rotatory eye movements mediated by the medial longitudinal fasciculus (MLF)
(D) project fibers directly to the striate cortex
(E) are concerned only with visual reflexes

5.9. The superior colliculus projects to all of the following, *except*:
(A) lateral posterior (LP)-pulvinar complex
(B) lateral geniculate body
(C) interstitial nucleus of Cajal
(D) reticular formation
(E) lumbar spinal cord

5.10. A patient exhibiting ipsilateral miosis, ptosis, and absence of facial sweating might have:
(A) Weber's syndrome
(B) neurosyphilis
(C) Horner's syndrome
(D) myasthenia gravis
(E) poliomyelitis

5.11. Loss of the pupillary light-reflex with preservation of the accommodation for near vision is characteristic of:
(A) Weber's syndrome
(B) multiple sclerosis
(C) capsular hemiplegia
(D) tabes dorsalis
(E) encephalitis

5.12. The electroencephalographic (EEG) arousal response:
(A) is dependent upon the integrity of the lemniscal system
(B) tends to synchronize electrocortical activity over broad cortical areas
(C) can be elicited only by specific tactile, visual, auditory, and olfactory stimuli
(D) is associated with desynchronization and activation of the cerebral cortex
(E) is not abolished by large lesions in the rostral midbrain tegmentum

5.13. Lesions of the midbrain tegmentum frequently are associated with:
(A) hypersomnia, muscular relaxation, slow respiration, and an EEG characterized by large amplitude slow waves
(B) unconsciousness, irregular respiration, and impaired cardiovascular function
(C) an EEG pattern similar to that associated with paradoxical sleep and rapid eye movements
(D) decerebrate rigidity and loss of thermoregulatory control
(E) increased muscle tone and collapse of the cardiovascular function

5.14. Ascending impulses in the brain stem reticular formation are conveyed:
(A) polysynaptically by chains of Golgi type II neurons
(B) by fibers of the medial longitudinal fasciculus
(C) by the central tegmental tract to parts of the intralaminar thalamic nuclei and hypothalamus
(D) from the pons and medulla directly to the cerebral cortex
(E) by the lemniscal systems

5.15. Barbiturate anesthesia:
(A) blocks transmission of impulses from peripheral receptors
(B) blocks transmission of impulses in the lemniscal systems
(C) depresses electrocortical activity selectively in sensory areas
(D) blocks synaptic transmission in the ascending reticular system
(E) depresses neural activity equally at all levels of the neuraxis

5.16. The principal ascending bundle arising from the medullary reticular formation:
(A) projects to the cerebellum
(B) is multisynaptic
(C) is the central tegmental fasciculus
(D) projects to the inferior olivary complex
(E) ascends in the periventricular and periaqueductal gray

5.17. The electroencephalographic (EEG) pattern seen in the cerveau isolé preparation:
- (A) resembles that of the awake state
- (B) is the same as that associated with paradoxical sleep
- (C) is the same as in the encéphale isolé preparation
- (D) reflects removal of the influences from the reticular formation upon electrocortical activity
- (E) demonstrates the importance of the lemniscal systems upon the EEG activity

5.18. The following are true concerning the red nucleus, *except*:
- (A) it receives projections from the interposed and dentate nuclei
- (B) it has a caudal magnocellular portion
- (C) it receives a somatotopic projection from the motor cortex
- (D) it sends uncrossed fibers to the inferior olive via the central tegmental tract
- (E) it projects uncrossed fibers to the intermediate zone (lamina VII) of the spinal gray

For each numbered item, select the one heading most closely associated with it. Each lettered heading may be selected once, more than once, or not at all.

Questions 5.19–5.22

- (A) Anesthetic state (barbiturates)
- (B) Slow wave sleep
- (C) Paradoxical (REM) sleep
- (D) Behavioral and EEG arousal response
- (E) Semicoma, hypersomnia, or akinetic mutism (coma vigil)

5.19. Associate with fast, low amplitude EEG activity, dreaming, bradycardia, and irregular respiration

5.20. Results from stimulation of most sensory receptors or stimulation of the brain stem reticular formation

5.21. Enhances neuronal conduction in the lemniscal systems and produces depression of synaptic conduction in the reticular formation

5.22. Associated with lesions in the midbrain reticular formation

For each numbered item, select the letter designating the part in Fig. 5.1 which matches it correctly. A lettered part may be selected once, more than once, or not at all.

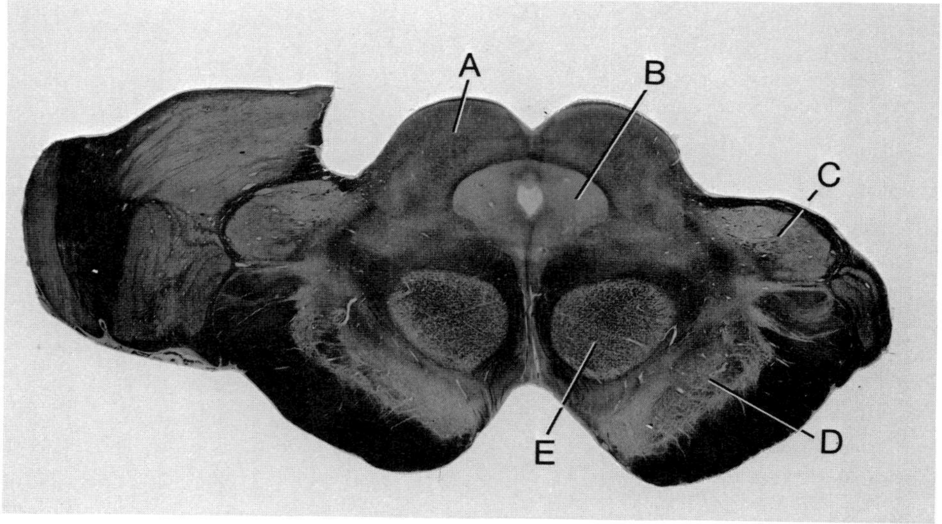

Figure 5.1. Transverse section of the brain stem.

5.23. Receives projections from the inferior colliculus

5.24. Has reciprocal connections with the parabigeminal nucleus

5.25. Projects descending fibers to the emboliform nucleus, the facial nucleus, the inferior olive, and the spinal cord

5.26. Cells of the same division project to thalamus and superior colliculus

For each numbered item, select the one heading most closely associated with it. Each lettered heading may be selected once, more than once, or not at all.

Questions 5.27–5.30

(A) Lesion in the optic nerve
(B) Lesion of oculomotor nerve
(C) Lesion of posterior commissure
(D) Lesion of superior cervical ganglion
(E) Lesion of facial nerve

5.27. Small pupil on side of lesion

5.28. No direct or consensual pupillary light reflex

5.29. Fully dilated pupil, ptosis, and no direct pupillary light reflex

5.30. Impaired ocular convergence

For each numbered item, select the letter designating the part in Fig. 5.2 which matches it correctly. A lettered part may be selected once, more than once, or not at all.

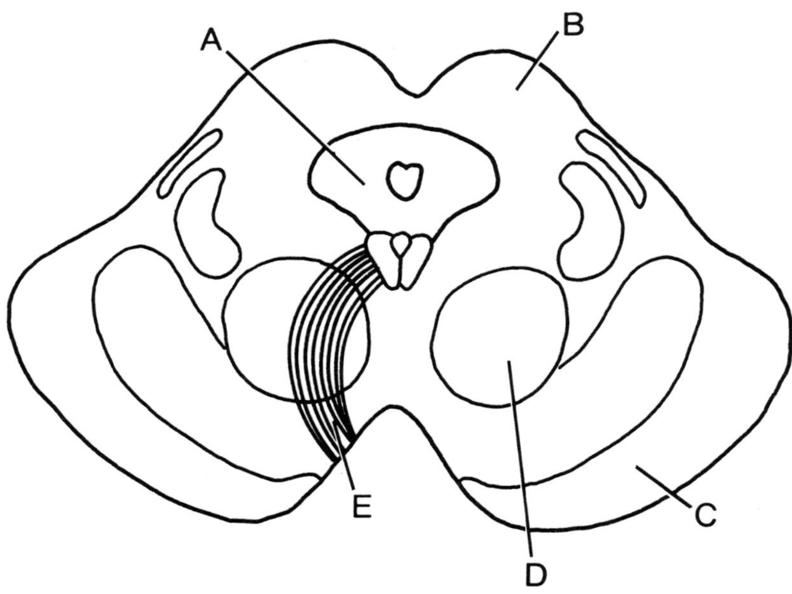

Figure 5.2

5.31. A lesion here would cause a unilateral ophthalmoplegia

5.32. Involved in generating tracking movements of the eyes and neck muscles

5.33. A lesion here would cause a contralateral diminution of flexor muscle tone

5.34. Implicated in nociceptive-suppressing pathways

For each numbered item, select the one heading most closely associated with it. Each lettered heading may be selected once, more than once, or not at all.

Questions 5.35–5.38

(A) Melatonin
(B) Serotonin
(C) Dopamine
(D) Substance P
(E) Acetylcholine

5.35. Substantia nigra pars compacta

5.36. Pineal body

5.37. Superior central nucleus

5.38. Trochlear nucleus

For each numbered item, select the letter designating the part in Fig. 5.3 which matches it correctly. A lettered part may be selected once, more than once, or not at all.

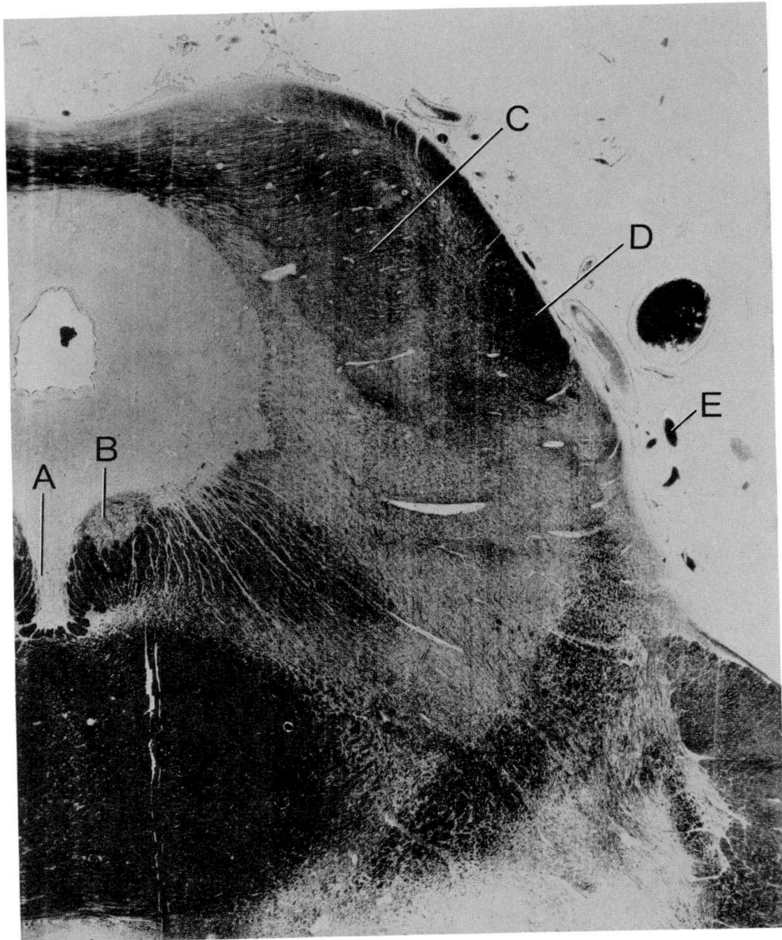

Figure 5.3. Photomicrograph of part of a transverse section through the mesencephalon.

5.39. A lesion here would produce predominantly vertical diplopia on left downward gaze

5.40. Projects serotonergic fibers to the substantia nigra and neostriatum

5.41. Tonotopically organized

5.42. Receives projections from the lateral lemniscus

For each numbered item, select the letter designating the part in Fig. 5.4 which matches it correctly. A lettered part may be selected once, more than once, or not at all.

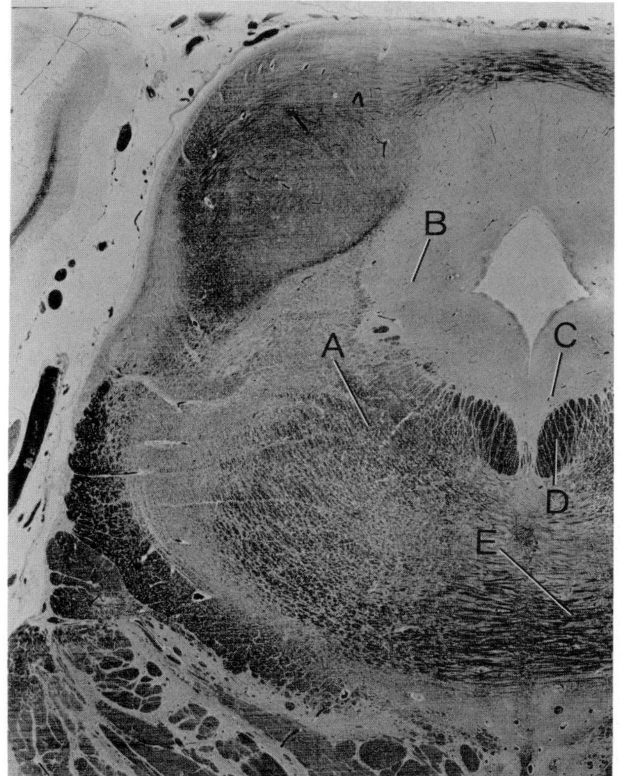

Figure 5.4. Photomicrograph of part of a transverse section through the mesencephalon.

5.43. Contains cerebellar projections to the contralateral thalamus

5.44. Contains uncrossed ascending fibers conveying gustatory sense

5.45. Descending spinal projections are concerned with analgesic mechanisms

5.46. Cells in this region distribute serotinergic fibers to the substantia nigra and neostriatum

For each numbered item, indicate whether it is associated with

A only (A)
B only (B)
Both A and B (C)
Neither A or B (D)

Questions 5.47–5.50

(A) Superficial layers of superior colliculus
(B) Deep layers of superior colliculus
(C) Both
(D) Neither

5.47. Anatomical organization resembles that of the cerebral cortex

5.48. Receives heterogenous inputs

5.49. Receives inputs from subcortical structures

5.50. Projects to the oculomotor nuclear complex

Questions 5.51–5.54

(A) Pupillary light reflex
(B) Accommodation-convergence reflex
(C) Both
(D) Neither

5.51. Involves optic nerve, optic tract, lateral geniculate body, and striate cortex

5.52. Involves corticofugal fibers from striate cortex

5.53. Involves efferent fibers from the pretectal olivary nucleus

5.54. Unaffected by a unilateral lesion in the striate cortex

Questions 5.55–5.59

(A) Vertical eye movements
(B) Horizontal eye movements
(C) Both
(D) Neither

5.55. Abducens nucleus

5.56. Interstitial nucleus of Cajal

5.57. Pontine paramedian reticular formation (PPRF)

5.58. Pretectal olivary nucleus

5.59. Rostral interstitial nucleus of the MLF (RiMLF)

For each numbered item in Fig. 5.5 indicate whether it is associated with

A only (A)
B only (B)
Both A and B (C)
Neither A nor B (D)
Shaded areas represent lesions.

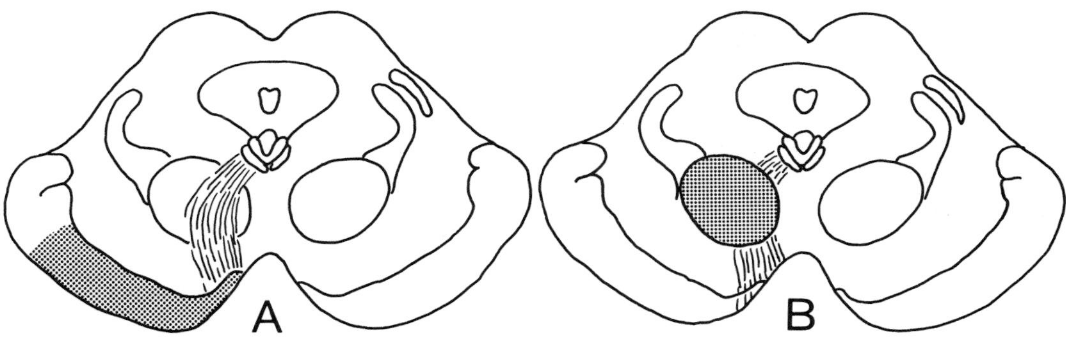

Figure 5.5

5.60. Cerebellar dyskinesia contralateral to lesion

5.61. Anisocoria, ptosis, and pupil unresponsive to light stimulus

5.62. Central type facial palsy contralateral to lesion

5.63. Ipsilateral cerebellar ataxia and tremor

For each numbered item, indicate whether it is associated with

A only (A)
B only (B)
Both A and B (C)
Neither A or B (D)

Questions 5.64–5.67

(A) Inferior cerebellar peduncle
(B) Superior cerebellar peduncle
(C) Both
(D) Neither

5.64. Transmits spinocerebellar fibers

5.65. Transmits efferents from deep cerebellar nuclei

5.66. Transmits olivocerebellar fibers

5.67. Transmits pontocerebellar fibers

For each of the incomplete statements below, *one* or *more* of the completions given is correct. Choose answer:

(A) Only **1, 2,** and **3** are correct
(B) Only **1** and **3** are correct
(C) Only **2** and **4** are correct
(D) Only **4** is correct
(E) **All** are correct

5.68. The trochlear nerve:
(1) conveys GVE fibers
(2) emerges dorsally from brain stem caudal to level of IV nucleus
(3) innervates the lateral rectus muscle
(4) decussates in the superior medullary velum

5.69. The rubrospinal tract:
(1) is somatotopically organized
(2) facilitates contralateral flexor muscle tone
(3) is synaptically linked with the ipsilateral cerebral cortex and the contralateral cerebellar paravermal cortex
(4) has terminations in the spinal gray which partially overlap those of the corticospinal tract

5.70. Tonotopic organization occurs in the following auditory relay structures:
(1) central nucleus of the inferior colliculus
(2) medial geniculate body
(3) transverse gyri of Heschl
(4) external nucleus of the inferior colliculus

5.71. Nuclei of the lateral or "sensory" reticular zone include:
(1) nucleus reticularis gigantocellularis
(2) nucleus reticularis parvicellularis
(3) nucleus reticularis pontis caudalis
(4) lateral reticular nucleus

5.72. The substantia nigra receives:
(1) serotonergic (5-HT) projections from the dorsal raphe nucleus
(2) strionigral fibers that have substance P (undecapeptide) as their neurotransmitter
(3) strionigral and pallidonigral projections that have GABA as their neurotransmitter
(4) dopaminergic fibers from the neostriatum

5.73. Fibers from raphe nuclei of the rostral brain stem:
(1) ascend in the medial forebrain bundle
(2) project to neostriatum
project to the hippocampus and amygdala
(4) project to the neocortex

5.74. *Direct* inputs to the oculomotor nuclear complex come from:
(1) the vestibular nuclei
(2) the frontal eye field
(3) the interstitial nucleus of Cajal
(4) the superior colliculus

5.75. The visceral nuclei of the oculomotor complex (Edinger-Westphal nuclei):
(1) project directly to spinal cord and a variety of brain stem nuclei
(2) are the site of lesions associated with the Argyll-Robertson pupil
(3) receive bilateral projections from the pretectal olivary nucleus
(4) receive information from the interstitial nucleus of Cajal involved in the accommodation reaction

5.76. The substantia nigra receives inputs from:
(1) the caudate and putamen
(2) the subthalamic nucleus
(3) the dorsal nucleus of the raphe
(4) the lateral pallidal segment

5.77. Electroencephalographic (EEG) desynchronization associated with behavioral arousal:
(1) is abolished in the encéphale isolé preparation
(2) is dependent on the integrity of the classic lemniscal pathways
(3) is maintained by activity in the midbrain raphe nuclei
(4) can be abolished by destruction of the central tegmental tract bilaterally

5.78. Projections from midbrain to spinal cord arise from:
(1) the superior colliculus
(2) the interstitial nucleus of Cajal
(3) the Edinger-Westphal nucleus
(4) the red nucleus

5.79. A lesion of the trochlear nerve may produce:
(1) predominantly vertical diplopia
(2) impaired ocular intorsion when the eye is abducted
(3) impaired downward motion when the eye is adducted
(4) horizontal diplopia

5.80. Visual accommodation:
(1) occurs automatically during ocular convergence
(2) is normally accompanied by pupillary constriction
(3) may persist although the pupillary light reflex has been abolished
(4) is dependent upon feedback from the striate cortex

5.81. The superior colliculus:
(1) receives primary visual input from the contralateral visual field
(2) has circular receptive fields of a concentric nature
(3) has cells which respond to movement of objects in the visual field which show directional selectivity
(4) has an uncrossed input from the striate cortex

5.82. The medullary reticular formation:
(1) is concerned primarily with inhibitory phenomena
(2) receives collateral fibers from all ascending systems and most sensory cranial nerve nuclei
(3) projects fibers to higher and lower levels of the neuraxis
(4) contains no cell groups projecting to the cerebellum

5.83. Paradoxical sleep:
(1) is associated with rapid eye movements
(2) is associated with dreaming
(3) may be triggered by neurons in the locus ceruleus
(4) is associated with small amplitude, desynchronized cortical activity

5.84. Repetitive stimulation of the midbrain reticular formation:
(1) gives rise to the electroencephalographic (EEG) arousal response
(2) gives rise to the recruiting response
(3) can block an on-going recruiting response
(4) causes hyperpolarization and depolarization of cortical dendrites which wax and wane

5.85. In a cerveau isolé preparation:
(1) the electroencephalogram (EEG) is characteristic of paradoxical sleep
(2) the EEG resembles that associated with "slow" sleep
(3) the EEG demonstrates the importance of the lemniscal system
(4) the EEG reflects the removal of the reticular activitating system upon electrocortical activity

Answers and Explanations*

5.1. **C** Although crossed and uncrossed axons from homonymous halves of the retinae reach the pretectum on one side, direct and consensual pupillary light reflexes depend upon bilateral pretectal projections to the visceral nuclei of the oculomotor complex. The most important nucleus is the pretectal olivary nucleus. See p. 185

5.2. **C** See Figs. 7-12 and 7-13

5.3. **C** Primary sensory neurons of the mesencephalic nucleus of cranial nerve V lie within the central nervous system. Only some of these cells are intermingled with those of the locus ceruleus. See p. 158

5.4. **C** A complete lesion of the oculomotor nerve results in ptosis, external strabismus and severe limitation of eye movements; the pupil is fully dilated and there is no direct pupillary light reflex. See p. 186

5.5. **C** Decerebrate rigidity is characterized by great increase in antigravity muscle tone; essentially γ rigidity. The resulting imbalance leaves facilitating mechanisms dominant. See p. 149

5.6. **D** Predominantly a vertical diplopia on attempted downward gaze to the opposite side. See p. 173

5.7. **B** A superior alternating hemiplegia (Weber's syndrome)

5.8. **A** See pp. 176–178

5.9. **E** Spinal projections from the superior colliculus are largely to cervical spinal segments

5.10. **C** A lesion involving sympathetic fibers. Such lesions can involve the brain stem, the cervical spinal cord or pre- or postganglionic cervical sympathetic fibers. See p. 186

5.11. **D** Argyll-Robertson pupil associated with central nervous system syphilis

5.12. **D** See pp. 189–190

5.13. **A** See p. 190

5.14. **C** The principal ascending bundle from the reticular formation of the pons and medulla is the central tegmental tract

5.15. **D** Barbiturate anesthesia blocks synaptic transmission in the reticular formation and depresses cortical activity in all regions

5.16. **C** See p. 190

5.17. **D** Represents transection of brain stem at midbrain level (cerveau isolé), while encéphale isolé is equivalent to a high spinal transection. See p. 189

5.18. **E** The rubrospinal tract is entirely crossed

5.19. **C** See pp. 167–168 and 388

5.20. **D** See pp. 189–190

5.21. **A** Barbiturates depress synaptic conduction in the brain stem reticular formation

5.22. **E** Such lesions destroy the ascending reticular activating system. See p. 190

5.23. **C** Medial geniculate body

5.24. **A** Superficial layers of the superior colliculus

5.25. **E** Red nucleus

5.26. **D** Applies to some cells of the pars reticulata of the substantia nigra (30–50%)

5.27. **D** Horner's syndrome

5.28. **A** Afferent limb of reflex arc is destroyed

5.29. **B** Complete lesion of cranial nerve III

* All page numbers and illustration citations refer to Carpenter: CORE TEXT OF NEUROANATOMY, 3rd edition; © 1985, Williams & Wilkins.

5.30. B Convergence is not possible with a complete oculomotor nerve lesion

5.31. E Oculomotor nerve

5.32. B Superior colliculus. See p. 179

5.33. D Red nucleus

5.34. A Periaqueductal gray

5.35. C See p. 225

5.36. A See p. 194

5.37. B See p. 166

5.38. E See p. 115

5.39. E Trochlear nerve

5.40. A Dorsal nucleus of raphe

5.41. C Central nucleus of inferior colliculus

5.42. C Inferior colliculus

5.43. E Decussation of superior cerebellar peduncle

5.44. A Central tegmental tract

5.45. B Periaqueductal gray

5.46. D Dorsal nucleus of raphe

5.47. A See p. 175

5.48. B See p. 176

5.49. C See p. 178

5.50. D See p. 179

5.51. B See p. 185

5.52. B

5.53. C See p. 185

5.54. D In the accommodation-convergence reflex, impulses from the striate cortex reach the ipsilateral superior colliculus and pretectum and are relayed via the pretectal olivary nucleus bilaterally to the visceral nuclei of the oculomotor complex

5.55. B The abducens nucleus, a center for conjugate horizontal eye movements, contains two populations of neurons: (1) those that form the abducens nerve and (2) internuclear neurons which ascend in the contralateral MLF to the medial rectus subdivision of the oculomotor complex. See pp. 153–154

5.56. A The interstitial nucleus of Cajal is concerned with rotatory and vertical eye movements. See p. 181 and Fig. 7-14

5.57. C The PPRF has output to both the abducens nucleus and the RiMLF. See pp. 154 and 185

5.58. D Pretectal olivary nucleus receives retinal afferents and projects bilaterally to visceral nuclei of the oculomotor complex. It is involved in pupillary light reflex

5.59. A RiMLF, located in Forel's field (junction of midbrain and diencephalon), is a center for vertical eye movements that receives input from the PPRF and vestibular nuclei. This nucleus projects ipsilaterally to oculomotor complex and is concerned primarily with downward eye movements. See pp. 154 and 185

5.60. B Lesion in region of red nucleus and superior cerebellar peduncle (syndrome of Benedikt). See p. 188

5.61. C Due to involvement of root fibers of oculomotor nerve

5.62. A Lesion in crus cerebri would involve corticobulbar fibers, including those projecting to the facial nucleus

5.63. D

5.64. C Fibers of the rostral spinocerebellar tract enter cerebellum by both peduncles. However, most spinocerebellar fibers are in the inferior cerebellar peduncle. See pp. 81–83

5.65. B See p. 211

5.66. A All olivocerebellar fibers traverse the contralateral inferior cerebellar peduncle

5.67. D These fibers form the middle cerebellar peduncle

5.68. C See pp. 163 and 173 and Figs. 6-26 and 7-5

5.69. E See pp. 186–187

5.70. A The external nucleus of the inferior colliculus is primarily involved in acousticomotor reflexes. See p. 173

5.71. C See p. 112

5.72. A Dopaminergic neurons are in the pars compacta of the substantia nigra and project to the striatum. See p. 191

5.73. E See pp. 166–167

5.74. B Of these structures only the vestibular nuclei and the interstitial nucleus of Cajal project directly to the oculomotor complex

5.75. B See pp. 95 and 185

5.76. **E** See pp. 192–194

5.77. **D** See p. 190

5.78. **E** All project fibers to spinal cord

5.79. **A** See p. 173

5.80. **E** In the Argyll-Robertson pupil, accommodation is preserved, but the light reflex is abolished. The mechanism for this is unknown

5.81. **E** See pp. 176–179

5.82. **B** See pp. 112–113 and 188

5.83. **E** See pp. 168 and 388

5.84. **B** See pp. 189 and 264

5.85. **C** See pp. 189 and 190

6

Cerebellum

Questions

Select the one best answer

6.1. The superior cerebellar peduncle contains:
- (A) fibers from the interposed nuclei which project to all parts of the opposite red nucleus
- (B) efferent fibers from all ipsilateral deep cerebellar nuclei and the anterior spinocerebellar tract
- (C) fibers from the dentate and interposed nuclei which project to parts of the opposite red nucleus and certain thalamic nuclei
- (D) Purkinje cell axons which convey inhibition
- (E) the anterior spinocerebellar tract and the uncinate fasciculus

6.2. Stimulation of the anterior interposed (emboliform) nucleus on one side:
- (A) increases ipsilateral flexor muscle tone
- (B) increases ipsilateral extensor muscle tone
- (C) diminishes muscle tone bilaterally
- (D) has no effect upon muscle tone
- (E) produces nystagmus

6.3. A cerebellar glomerulus:
- (A) consists of two different presynaptic elements and one type of postsynaptic element
- (B) is found only in cerebellar islands close to Golgi type II cells
- (C) has a core composed of several mossy fiber rosettes
- (D) is isolated from Purkinje cells by a glia lamella
- (E) gives rise to a single axon that contacts the smooth branchlets of Purkinje cells

6.4. The cerebellar cortex has been compared with a computer because it:
- (A) stores information for later retrieval
- (B) has complex intracortical circuits that modify sensory input
- (C) processes inputs from virtually all sensory systems and provides a clear and quick response
- (D) processes information rapidly and has dynamic memory
- (E) functions by feedback mechanisms

6.5. Paravermal regions of the cerebellar cortex project fibers ipsilaterally to:
- (A) emboliform and fastigial nuclei
- (B) dentate and fastigial nuclei
- (C) globose and emboliform nuclei
- (D) fastigial and globose nuclei
- (E) dentate nucleus

6.6. All of the following are cerebellar cortical neurons, *except*:
- (A) Golgi type II cells
- (B) basket cells
- (C) outer stellate cells
- (D) granule cells
- (E) Bergmann cells

6.7. Lesions of the dentate nucleus or superior cerebellar peduncle may produce all of the following, *except*:
- (A) decomposition of movement
- (B) tremor during movement
- (C) dysmetria
- (D) exaggerated myotactic reflexes
- (E) ataxia

6.8. The output of the cerebellar cortex:
(A) consists of Purkinje cell axons that emerge via the superior cerebellar peduncle
(B) is excitatory to the deep cerebellar nuclei
(C) exerts inhibitory influences upon the deep cerebellar nuclei and the lateral vestibular nucleus
(D) projects in three longitudinally organized zones to the globose, emboliform, and dentate nuclei
(E) is ipsilateral in the hemisphere and partially crossed in the vermis

6.9. That portion of the cerebellar cortex especially concerned with processing auditory and visual signals is the:
(A) anterior lobe
(B) paramedian lobule
(C) ansiform lobule
(D) flocculonodular lobule
(E) simple lobule, folium, and tuber

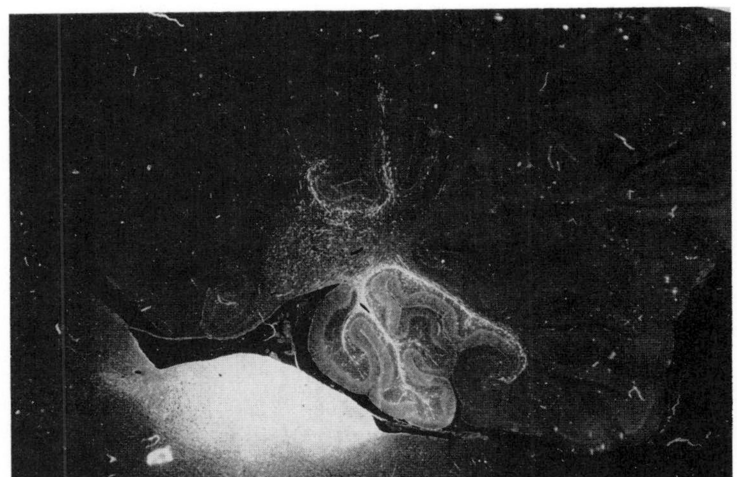

Figure 6.1. Autoradiograph of a sagittal section of the monkey cerebellum.

6.10. The part of the cerebellum containing the most densely labeled afferent fibers in Fig. 6.1 represents the:

(A) paleocerebellum
(B) neocerebellum
(C) paramedian lobule
(D) flocculus and uvula
(E) nodulus and uvula

6.11. All of the following are precerebellar nuclei, *except*:
(A) perihypoglossal nuclei
(B) lateral reticular nucleus
(C) reticulotegmental nucleus
(D) spinal trigeminal nucleus
(E) oculomotor nucleus

For each numbered item, select the one heading most closely associated with it. Each lettered heading may be selected once, more than once, or not at all.

Questions 6.12–6.15

(A) Dentate nucleus
(B) Interposed nuclei
(C) Fastigial nucleus
(D) Cerebellovestibular projections
(E) Uncinate fasciculus

6.12. Receive(s) Purkinje cell axons from all parts of the ipsilateral cerebellar vermis

6.13. Arise(s) somatotopically from the anterior lobe vermis

6.14. Receive(s) and projects collaterals to the lateral zone of the cerebellar cortex

6.15. Project(s) somatotopically upon cells in caudal parts of the opposite red nucleus

Questions 6.16–6.19

(A) Basket cell axons
(B) Climbing fibers
(C) Outer stellate cells
(D) Golgi cell axons
(E) Parallel fibers

6.16. Do not contact Purkinje cells

6.17. Synapse on Purkinje cell spiny branchlets

6.18. Synapse on the Purkinje cell soma

6.19. Synapse on smooth dendritic branchlets of Purkinje cells

Questions 6.20–6.23

(A) Ablation of the anterior lobe of cerebellum
(B) Stimulation of anterior lobe of cerebellum
(C) Ablation of archicerebellum
(D) Lesions of the dentate nucleus
(E) Lesions of neocerebellar cortex of the hemisphere

6.20. May increase or decrease ipsilateral muscle tone

6.21. Associated with ataxia and disturbances of equilibrium

6.22. Produces an increase in muscle tone by removal of inhibitory influences

6.23. May produce transient, or only minimal, disturbances of motor activities

For each numbered item, select the letter designating the part in Fig. 6.2 which matches it correctly. A lettered part may be selected once, more than once, or not at all.

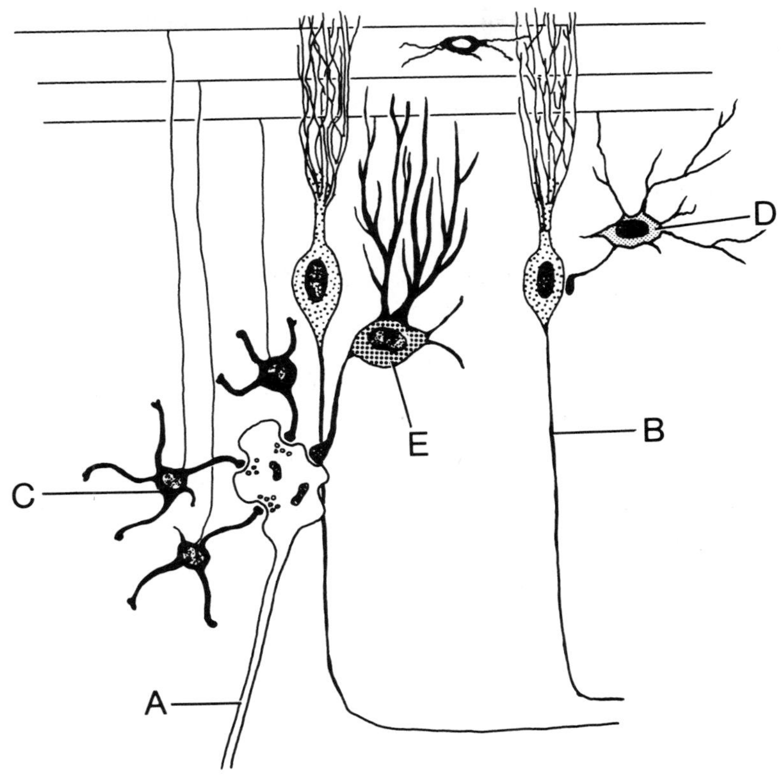

Figure 6.2

6.24. Conveys excitatory input to the cerebellar cortex

6.25. Forms terminal arborizations about somata of many Purkinje cells

6.26. Forms "crossover" synapses with Purkinje cell dendrites

6.27. Establishes synaptic contact with the deep cerebellar nuclei

Questions 6.28–6.31

(A) Pontocerebellar fibers
(B) Olivocerebellar fibers
(C) Reticulocerebellar fibers
(D) Vestibulocerebellar fibers
(E) Noradrenergic cerebellar afferents

6.28. Terminate around Purkinje cell somata

6.29. Arise from a peripheral ganglion and brain stem relay nuclei

6.30. Most massive cerebellar afferent system

6.31. Synapse on smooth branchlets of Purkinje cell dendrites

For each numbered item, select the letter designating the part in Fig. 6.3 which matches it correctly. A lettered part may be selected once, more than once, or not at all.

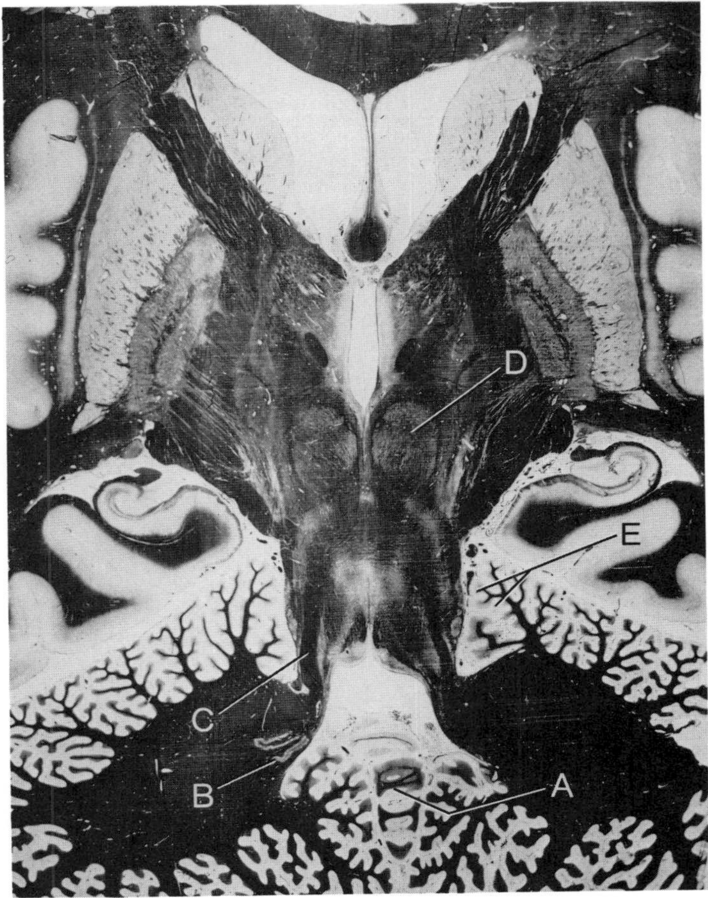

Figure 6.3. Horizontal section in the axis of the brain stem through the cerebellum, midbrain, and diencephalon. (From H. A. Riley, *Atlas of the Basal Ganglia, Brain Stem and Spinal Cord*, 1943; courtesy of Williams & Wilkins, Baltimore.)

6.32. Stimulation of this region can inhibit extensor muscle tone ipsilaterally

6.33. Represents the major cerebellar efferent pathway

6.34. Purkinje cells project to the fastigial nucleus

6.35. Different parts receive terminals or collaterals from the contralateral dentate, emboliform, and globose nuclei

For each numbered item, select the one heading most closely associated with it. Each lettered heading may be selected once, more than once, or not at all.

Questions 6.36–6.39

(A) Climbing fibers
(B) Mossy fibers
(C) Both
(D) Neither

6.36. Excitatory actions upon Purkinje cells

6.37. Pontocerebellar projection

6.38. “Cross-over” synapse

6.39. Convey “sensory inputs” to cerebellar cortex

For each numbered item in Fig. 6.4, indicate whether it is associated with

A only (A)
B only (B)
Both A and B (C)
Neither A nor B (D)

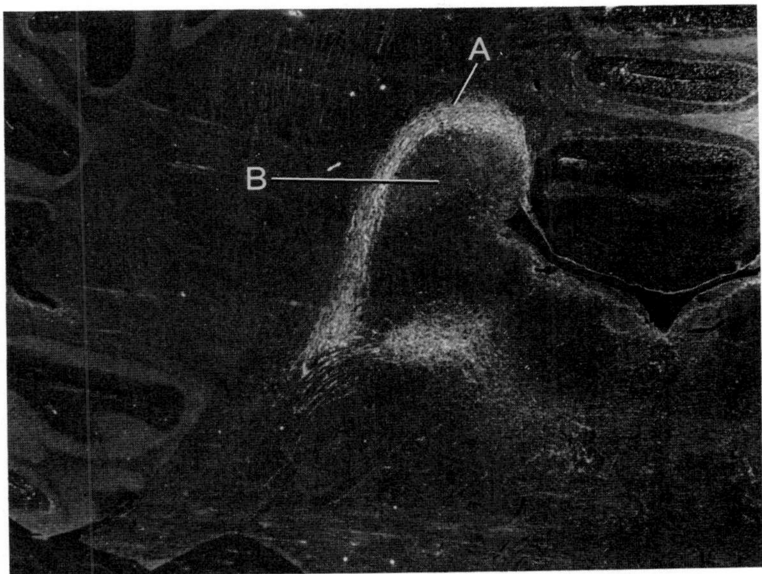

Figure 6.4. Photomicrograph of a transverse autoradiograph taken at a rostral pontine level. Fibers of one cerebellar efferent pathway are labeled. (From M. B. Carpenter, *Core Text of Neuroanatomy*, 1985; courtesy of Williams & Wilkins, Baltimore.)

6.40. Fibers cross within cerebellum

6.41. Fibers originate from all ipsilateral deep cerebellar nuclei

6.42. Fibers have terminations in all parts of contralateral red nucleus

6.43. GABAergic fibers

For each numbered item, indicate whether it is associated with

A only (A)
B only (B)
Both A and B (C)
Neither A or B (D)

Questions 6.44–6.47

(A) Anterior lobe of cerebellum
(B) Flocculonodular lobule
(C) Both
(D) Neither

6.44. Stimulation can modify ipsilateral extensor muscle tone

6.45. Receives serotonergic fibers from the raphe nuclei

6.46. Receive somatotopically organized inputs from stretch receptors

6.47. Can exert inhibitory influences upon vestibular nuclei via Purkinje cell axons

Questions 6.48–6.51

(A) Purkinje cells
(B) Fastigial nucleus
(C) Both
(D) Neither

6.48. Projects bilaterally and fairly symmetrically upon the lateral and inferior vestibular nuclei

6.49. Gamma (α)-aminobutyric acid

6.50. Excitatory influences conveyed to nuclei at all levels of the brain stem

6.51. Direct inhibition of cells in the ipsilateral lateral vestibular nucleus

For each of the incomplete statements below, *one* or *more* of the completions given is correct. Choose answer:

(A) Only **1, 2,** and **3** are correct
(B) Only **1** and **3** are correct
(C) Only **2** and **4** are correct
(D) Only **4** is correct
(E) **All** are correct

6.52. Climbing fibers in the cerebellum:
(1) arise from cells of the inferior olivary complex
(2) exert "all or none" excitatory effects upon Purkinje cells
(3) terminate on smooth branchlets of Purkinje cell dendrites
(4) project to all parts of the cerebellar cortex and to all deep cerebellar nuclei

6.53. A cerebellar glomerulus is a synaptic complex formed by:
(1) a single mossy fiber rosette
(2) axon terminals of Golgi II cells
(3) dendritic endings of granule cells
(4) climbing fibers

6.54. Fastigial efferent fibers emerge from the cerebellum via the:

(1) superior cerebellar peduncle
(2) uncinate fasciculus
(3) middle cerebellar peduncle
(4) juxtarestiform body

6.55. In the neocerebellar syndrome:

(1) truncal ataxia is the most prominent feature
(2) tremor, ataxia, and asynergic phenomenon occur as a constellation of disturbances
(3) motor disturbances occur at rest
(4) motor disturbances undergo an attenuation in time

6.56. Fibers or collaterals of the dentate nucleus terminate contralaterally in the:

(1) ventral lateral (VLc) and ventral posterolateral (VPLo) thalamic nuclei
(2) rostral intralaminar thalamic nuclei
(3) reticular nuclei of the brain stem
(4) parvicellular red nucleus

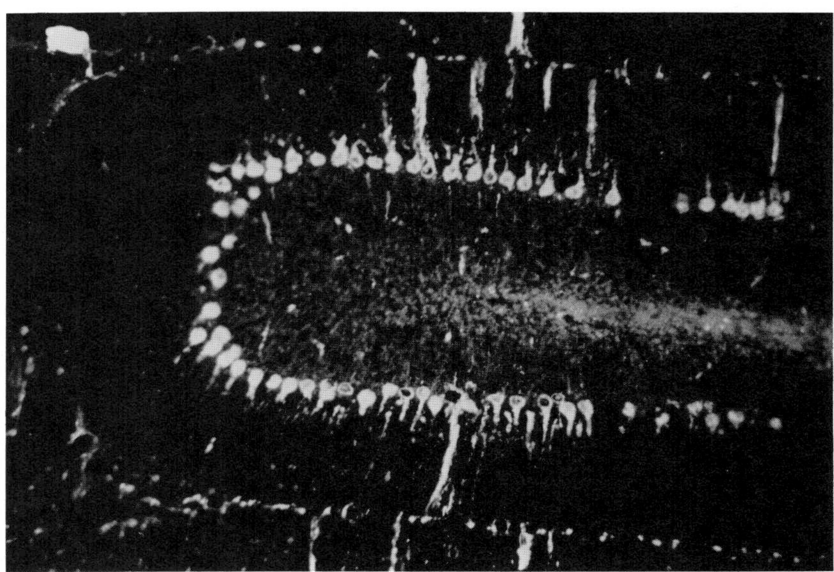

Figure 6.5

6.57. The HRP labeled cells in a dark field photomicrograph of the cerebellar cortex in Fig. 6.5:

(1) receive excitatory inputs from climbing and mossy fibers
(2) have GABA as their neurotransmitter
(3) receive inhibitory inputs only via basket cells
(4) project to the deep cerebellar nuclei in a topographic fashion

6.58. The cerebellum exerts its influences at segmental levels of the neuraxis via:

(1) paravermal cortex → emboliform nucleus → red nucleus → rubrospinal tract
(2) vermal cortex → fastigial nucleus → lateral vestibular nucleus → vestibulospinal tract
(3) lateral hemispheric cortex → dentate nucleus → ventral lateral (VLc) and ventral posterolateral (VPLo) thalamic nuclei → corticospinal tract
(4) anterior vermal cortex → lateral vestibular nucleus → vestibulospinal tract

6.59. Cerebellar influences upon motor activities are exerted ipsilaterally, because:

(1) projections from the emboliform nucleus and the red nucleus are both crossed
(2) fastigial efferent projections are mainly crossed
(3) dentatothalamic and corticospinal fibers are mainly crossed
(4) cortical projections to the deep cerebellar nuclei are ipsilateral

6.60. The cerebellum, consisting of three lobes, is divided by five fissures, so that:

(1) the posterior lobe lies caudal to the primary fissure
(2) the flocculonodular lobule lies caudal to the posterolateral fissure
(3) the horizontal fissure divides the posterior lobe into crus I and crus II
(4) the simple lobule is the most caudal part of the anterior lobe

6.61. Sensory input to the cerebellar cortex:

(1) is somatotopically organized in the ipsilateral anterior lobe and bilaterally in the paramedian lobules
(2) includes tactile sense, audition, and vision
(3) is conveyed primarily via the inferior and middle cerebellar peduncles
(4) includes impulses from pressure and stretch receptors

6.62. The most massive inputs to the cerebellar cortex arise from the:

(1) pontine nuclei
(2) reticular formation
(3) inferior olivary nuclear complex
(4) spinocerebellar systems

6.63. The inferior olivary nuclear complex:

(1) receives descending fibers via the central tegmental tract that terminate in parts of the principal nucleus
(2) receives ascending spinal fibers that terminate in the accessory olivary nuclei
(3) gives rise to crossed climbing fibers
(4) projects to all deep cerebellar nuclei

6.64. The cerebellum is:

(1) derived from ectodermal thickening about the rostral borders of the fourth ventricle
(2) receives inputs from virtually all types of receptors
(3) concerned with equilibrium, regulation of muscle tone, and coordination of motor function
(4) exerts its major influences upon motor function automatically, and indirectly via brain stem relay nuclei

6.65. Cerebellar dyskinesia

(1) most commonly is associated with lesions involving the deep cerebellar nuclei
(2) involves only coordinated voluntary or associated movements
(3) when due to a nonprogressive lesion, tends in time to become less severe
(4) rarely is associated with disturbances of speech

Answers and Explanations*

6.1. **C** All deep cerebellar nuclei, except the fastigial nucleus, project fibers to parts of the contralateral red nucleus and to the so-called "cell sparse zone" of the ventral lateral thalamus nucleus (VLc, area X and VPLo). See pp. 211–214

6.2. **A** The emboliform nucleus is somatotopically linked to cells of contralateral red nucleus, which in turn give rise to crossed rubrospinal fibers exerting a facilitatory influence upon flexor muscle tone. See pp. 213–214

6.3. **A** See p. 204

6.4. **C** See p. 219

6.5. **C** Paraventral cortex projects to the interposed nuclei which project fibers via the superior cerebellar peduncle; collaterals project back to the paravermal cortex. See pp. 208–209

6.6. **E** Bergmann cells are modified astrocytes that lie in a satellite formation around Purkinje cells

6.7. **D** Such lesions usually are associated with very sluggish or absent deep tendon reflexes and diminished muscle tone

6.8. **C** The entire output of the cerebellar cortex is via Purkinje cell axons which have GABA as their neurotransmitter. See p. 207

6.9. **E** See p. 210 and Fig. 8-12

6.10. **E** Primary vestibular projections to the granular layer of the nodulus and parts of the uvula

6.11. **E**

6.12. **C** In this strictly unilateral projection Purkinje cell axons from various vermal lobules terminate in nearest region of the fastigial nucleus

6.13. **D** Somatotopically organized cerebellovestibular fibers from the anterior lobe vermis project mainly to the lateral vestibular nucleus. See p. 216

6.14. **A** See pp. 208–209

6.15. **B** See p. 213

6.16. **D** Golgi cell axons terminate in cerebellar glomeruli

6.17. **E** Parallel fibers representing the terminate portions of granule cell axons

6.18. **A** Basket cell axons arborize in a terminal fashion about the somata of 8–10 Purkinje cells. See p. 201

6.19. **B** Climbing fibers, originating from cells in the inferior olivary nuclear complex, synapse upon smooth branchlets of Purkinje cell dendrites and have "all or none" excitatory drives. See p. 205

6.20. **B** Effect depends upon parameters of stimulus. Low frequency stimulation (2–10 Hz) increases extensor muscle tone, while frequencies of 30–300 Hz diminish muscle tone. See p. 219

6.21. **C** See p. 219

6.22. **A** Ablations of the anterior lobe cortex remove inhibitory influences acting upon the vestibular nuclei

6.23. **E** Lesions of the neocerebellar cortex, if not massive, produce minimal disturbances

6.24. **C** Parallel fiber, representing an axon of granule cell

6.25. **D** Basket cell

6.26. **C** Parallel fibers

6.27. **B** Purkinje cell axon

6.28. **E** See p. 206

6.29. **D** Arise from the vestibular ganglion and nuclei

* All page numbers and illustration citations refer to Carpenter: CORE TEXT OF NEUROANATOMY, 3rd edition; © 1985, Williams & Wilkins.

6.30. **A** Largest system of cerebellar afferent fibers

6.31. **B** Climbing fibers

6.32. **E** Anterior lobe of cerebellum

6.33. **C** Superior cerebellar peduncle

6.34. **A** Cerebellar vermis

6.35. **D** Red nucleus

6.36. **A**

6.37. **B**

6.38. **D** Parallel fibers arise from granule cells

6.39. **B** Most "sensory inputs," including those conveyed by pontocerebellar fibers, terminate as mossy fibers

6.40. **A** Uncinate fasciculus

6.41. **D**

6.42. **B** Superior cerebellar peduncle

6.43. **D**

6.44. **A** Different parameters of stimulation can increase or decrease extensor muscle tone

6.45. **C** Serotonergic fibers are distributed to all layers in all parts of the cerebellar cortex

6.46. **A** Spinocerebellar systems terminate somatotopically in the anterior lobe

6.47. **C** Output via Purkinje cells has an inhibitory action

6.48. **B** See p. 214

6.49. **A** Neurotransmitter of Purkinje cells

6.50. **B** Fibers are distributed to nuclei at all levels of the brain stem

6.51. **A** Purkinje cells in the anterior lobe project ipsilaterally to the lateral vestibular nucleus

6.52. **E** See p. 209

6.53. **A** See p. 204

6.54. **C** See p. 214

6.55. **C** See p. 218

6.56. **E** See pp. 211–212

6.57. **C** The retrograde label is in Purkinje cells

6.58. **E** All represent pathways by which cerebellar influences are distributed in the neuraxis

6.59. **B** Cerebellar influences upon muscle tone are exerted via the rubrospinal (flexor tone) and vestibulospinal (extensor tone) tracts. Coordination of motor function involves cerebellar influences on the motor cortex exerted via thalamic nuclei

6.60. **B** The flocculonodular lobule lies rostral to the posterolateral fissure. The simple lobule is immediately caudal to the primary fissure and is not part of the anterior lobe of the cerebellum

6.61. **E** See p. 210

6.62. **B** The pontine nuclei give rise to mainly crossed fibers of the middle cerebellar peduncle, the largest single group of cerebellar afferents. The inferior olivary complex gives rise to crossed olivocerebellar fibers, the largest component of the inferior cerebellar peduncle.

6.63. **E** See pp. 111–112 and 209

6.64. **E** The cerebellum is derived from the rhombic lip which lies dorsal to the sulcus limitans and exerts its major influences upon motor functions indirectly via brain stem nuclei

6.65. **A** Speech disturbances are common with chronic neocerebellar lesions

7

Diencephalon and Thalamus

Questions

Select the one best answer

7.1. A patient with a right homonymous hemianopsia and congruent field defects, most likely has a lesion of the:
- (A) left optic tract
- (B) left striate cortex
- (C) right lateral geniculate body
- (D) left superior colliculus
- (E) right optic radiation

7.2. A lesion in Meyer's loop (i.e., geniculocalcarine fibers in the temporal lobe) on the right side would produce:
- (A) left homonymous hemianopsia
- (B) left inferior homonymous quadrantic visual field defect
- (C) left superior homonymous quadrantanopsia
- (D) a visual field defect in the left superior temporal quadrant
- (E) bitemporal quadrantanopsia

7.3. After a long period, enucleation of the left eye would produce transneuronal degeneration:
- (A) bilaterally in the striate cortex
- (B) in the right striate cortex
- (C) in the right superior colliculus
- (D) in complementary layers of the lateral geniculate body bilaterally
- (E) in the parvicellular layers of the lateral geniculate body bilaterally

7.4. The lesion producing a bitemporal hemianopsia involves:
- (A) both optic nerves
- (B) both optic tracts
- (C) crossing fibers in the optic chiasm
- (D) the primary visual cortex
- (E) the lateral geniculate bodies

7.5. Transneuronal degeneration from a midsagittal section of the optic chiasm would involve cells:
- (A) only in the ventral lateral geniculate nucleus
- (B) only in the dorsal lateral geniculate nucleus
- (C) in the bilaminar segment of the lateral geniculate bilaterally
- (D) in all layers of the lateral geniculate body
- (E) in the pretectum

7.6. Neurons in the ventral lateral geniculate nucleus:
- (A) project primarily to cortical areas 18 and 19
- (B) project to the pretectum, the superior colliculus and the suprachiasmatic nucleus
- (C) receive a binocular retinal input
- (D) project to cortical area 17
- (E) are derivatives of the dorsal thalamus

7.7. Melatonin production by the pineal gland:
- (A) is regulated by neuronal output from the raphe nuclei of the midbrain
- (B) is abolished when the optic tract is severed
- (C) is abolished when the optic nerve is severed
- (D) continues to be produced in circadian fashion under conditions of constant darkness
- (E) tends to be increased during hours of light

7.8. The inhibitory surround (periphery) of the receptive field of a ganglion cell of the retina is most likely to have the following anatomical substrate:

(A) linkage of rods and cones to bipolar cells to amacrine cells
(B) linkage of rods to bipolar cells to ganglion cells
(C) linkage of cones to bipolar cells to ganglion cells
(D) linkage of rods and cones to bipolar cells and ganglion cells
(E) linkage of rods, horizontal cells, and ganglion cells

7.9. All of the following characterize the thalamus, or parts of it, *except*:

(A) extends from the region of the interventricular foramen to the posterior commissure
(B) all nuclear subdivisions lie medial to the internal capsule
(C) the pulvinar constitutes the largest subdivision
(D) is separated from the hypothalamus by the hypothalamic sulcus
(E) the reticular nucleus of the thalamus lies between the external medullary lamina and the internal capsule

7.10. The intralaminar thalamic nuclei which receive the largest input from the neocortex are:

(A) the paracentral and central lateral nuclei
(B) reticular nuclei of the thalamus
(C) centromedian and parafascicularis nuclei
(D) the periventricular nuclei
(E) central medial and central lateral nuclei

For each numbered item, select the one heading most closely associated with it. Each lettered heading may be selected once, more than once, or not at all.

Questions 7.11–7.14

(A) Anterior limb of internal capsule
(B) Posterior limb of internal capsule
(C) Retrolenticular internal capsule
(D) Sublenticular part of internal capsule
(E) Genu of the internal capsule

7.11. Contains superior thalamic radiation

7.12. Contains corticobulbar fibers

7.13. Auditory radiation

7.14. Frontopontine fibers

Questions 7.15–7.18

(A) Ventral posterior inferior (VPI) nucleus
(B) Medial geniculate nucleus (MG)
(C) Ventral posteromedial (VPM) nucleus
(D) Ventral lateral nucleus, pars caudalis (VPLc)
(E) Ventral posteromedial, pars parvicellularis (VPMpc)

7.15. Ventral laminated part projects to primary auditory cortex

7.16. Receives uncrossed ascending special visceral afferent input

7.17. Receives afferent input from most of the cranial dura mater

7.18. Receives terminals of medial lemniscus and spinothalamic tracts

For each numbered item, select the lettered part in Fig. 7.1 most closely associated with it. Each letter may be selected once, more than once, or not at all.

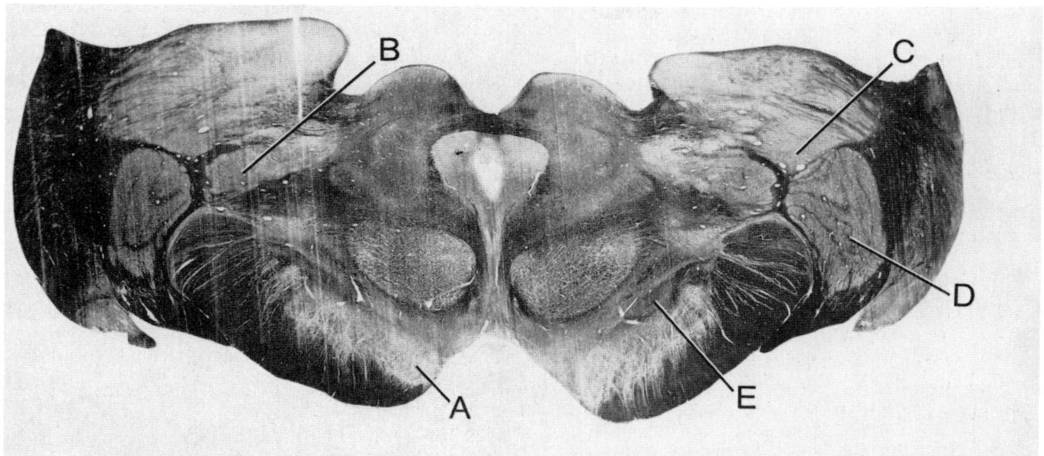

Figure 7.1. Transverse section through the rostral midbrain and caudal diencephalon. (From M. B. Carpenter, *Core Text of Neuroanatomy*, 1985; courtesy of Williams & Wilkins, Baltimore.)

7.19. Involved in linkage of extrageniculate visual system

7.20. Afferents project via brachium of the inferior colliculus

7.21. One cytological subdivision of this nucleus has cells which project dichotomizing axons to thalamus and superior colliculus

7.22. Ventral division of nucleus has only subcortical projections

For each numbered item, select the one heading most closely associated with it. Each lettered heading may be selected once, more than once, or not at all.

Questions 7.23–7.26

(A) Dorsomedial nucleus
(B) Ventral anterior nucleus
(C) Ventral posterolateral nucleus, pars oralis (VPLo)
(D) Ventral posterolateral nucleus pars caudalis (VPLc)
(E) Inferior and lateral pulvinar

7.23. Involved in extrageniculate visual pathways

7.24. Projects to primary (S I) and secondary (SS II) somesthetic areas

7.25. Has properties of specific and nonspecific thalamic nuclei

7.26. Projects to frontal lobe rostral to premotor area

For each numbered item, select the lettered lesion area (*vertical lines*) most closely associated with it in Fig. 7.2. Each letter may be selected once, more than once, or not at all.

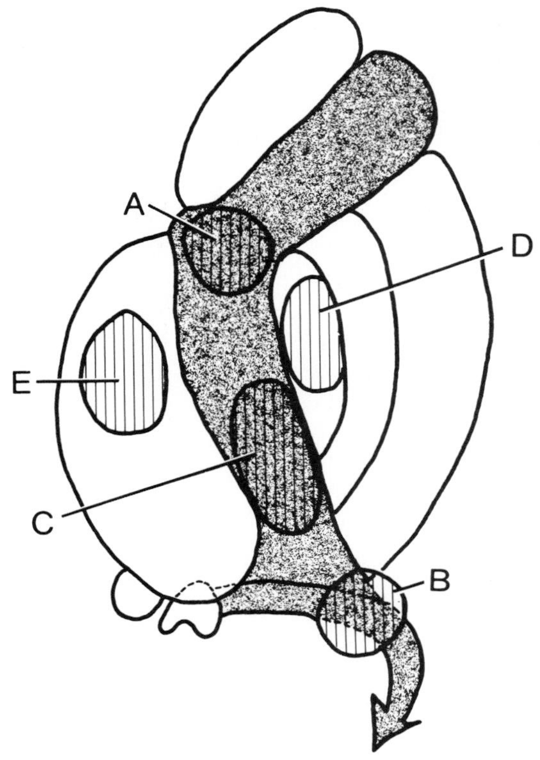

Figure 7.2

7.27. Homonymous hemianopsia

7.28. Contralateral hemiparesis

7.29. Central type facial paresis

7.30. Personality change

For each numbered item, select the lettered part in Fig. 7.3 most closely associated with it. Each letter may be selected once, more than once, or not at all.

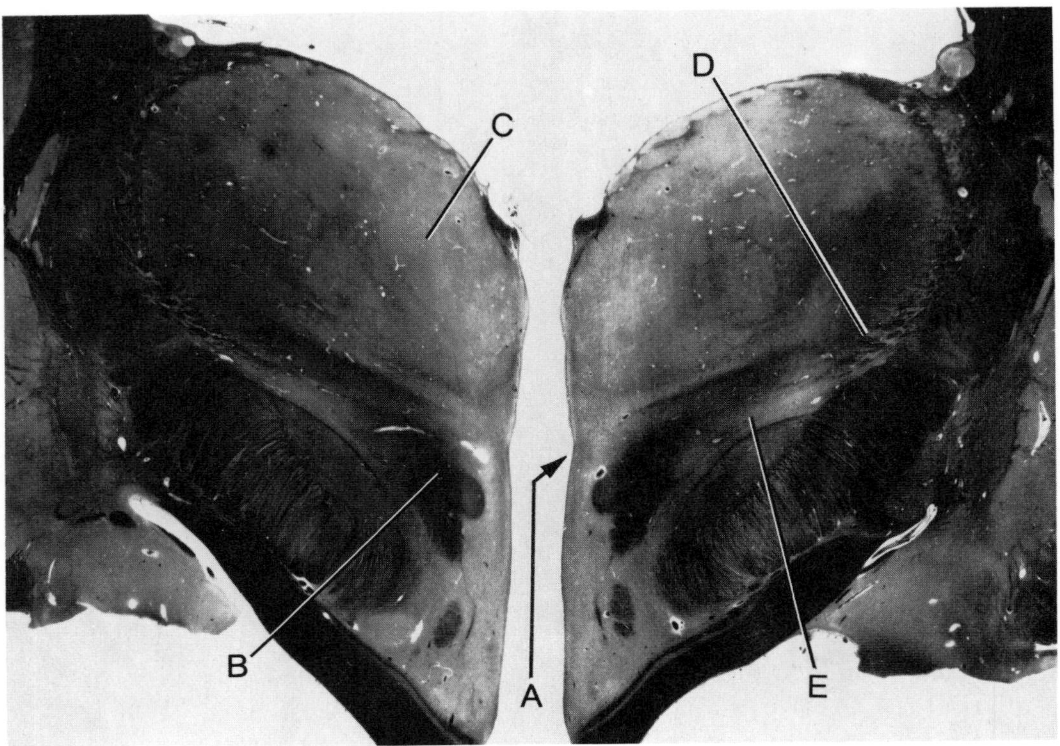

Figure 7.3. Transverse section through the diencephalon and corpus striatum. (From M. B. Carpenter, *Core Text of Neuroanatomy*, 1985; courtesy of Williams & Wilkins, Baltimore.)

7.31. Separates fibers of the lenticular fasciculus and thalamic fasciculus

7.32. Largest component of the ventrobasal nuclear complex

7.33. Separates thalamus and hypothalamus

7.34. Forel's field H

For each numbered item, select the one heading most closely associated with it. Each lettered heading may be selected once, more than once, or not at all.

Questions 7.35–7.38
Thalamic Nuclei

(A) Specific sensory relay nuclei
(B) Cortical relay nuclei
(C) Association nuclei
(D) Intralaminar nuclei
(E) Subcortical projection nuclei

7.35. Project to broad regions of the frontal, parietal temporal, and occipital cortex

7.36. Topographically or somatotopically organized, place and modality specific and synaptically secure

7.37. Receive inputs from the deep cerebellar nuclei, the globus pallidus, hypothalamus and the hippocampal formation

7.38. Project to the striatum and broad regions of the frontal and parietal cortex

For each numbered item select the lettered lesion most closely associated with it in Fig. 7.4. Each letter may be selected once, more than once, or not at all.

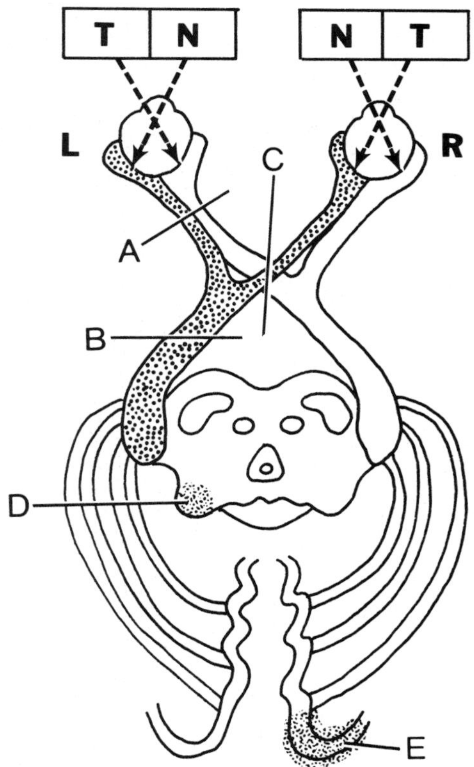

Figure 7.4. Schematic diagram of the visual pathways. *A, B, C, D,* and *E* are the sites of lesions. *T* and *N* refer to temporal and nasal halves of the visual field and *L* and *R* indicate left and right. (From M. B. Carpenter, *Core Text of Neuroanatomy*, 1985; courtesy of Williams & Wilkins, Baltimore.)

Questions 7.39–7.42

(A) Lesion at A
(B) Lesion at B
(C) Lesion at C
(D) Lesion at D
(E) Lesion at E

7.39. Would produce a left homonymous hemianopsia

7.40. Would abolish both direct and consensual pupillary light reflexes

7.41. Would after a long period of time produce transneuronal degeneration in the same three layers of each lateral geniculate body

7.42. Would produce cellular degeneration in parvicellular layers of the ipsilateral lateral geniculate body

For each numbered item select the lettered structure most closely associated with it in Fig. 7.5. Each letter may be selected once, more than once, or not at all.

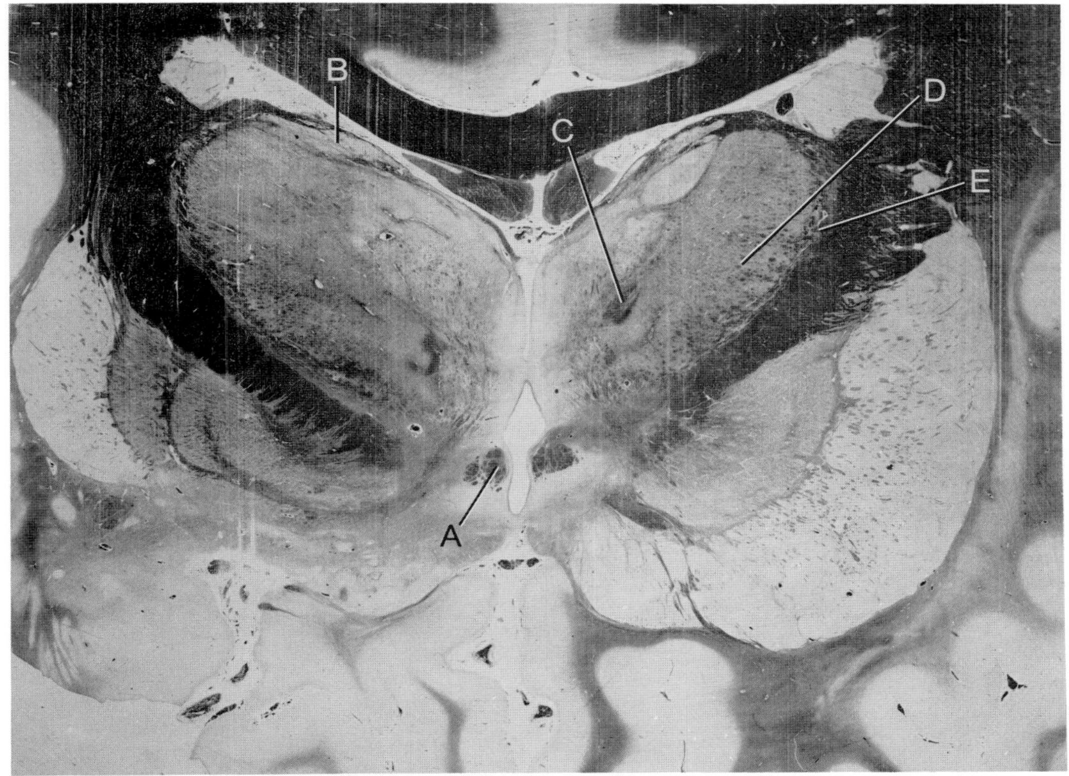

Figure 7.5. Transverse section through the diencephalon and corpus striatum. (From H. A. Riley, *Atlas of the Basal Ganglia, Brain Stem and Spinal Cord,* 1943; courtesy of Williams & Wilkins.)

7.43. Receives cortical afferents and collaterals of efferents from other thalamic nuclei, but has no cortical projection

7.44. Pars oralis receives output from medial pallidal segment

7.45. Association nucleus of thalamus

7.46. Contains fibers from mammillary nuclei

For each numbered item, select the lettered structure most closely associated with it in Fig. 7.6. Each letter may be selected once, more than once, or not at all.

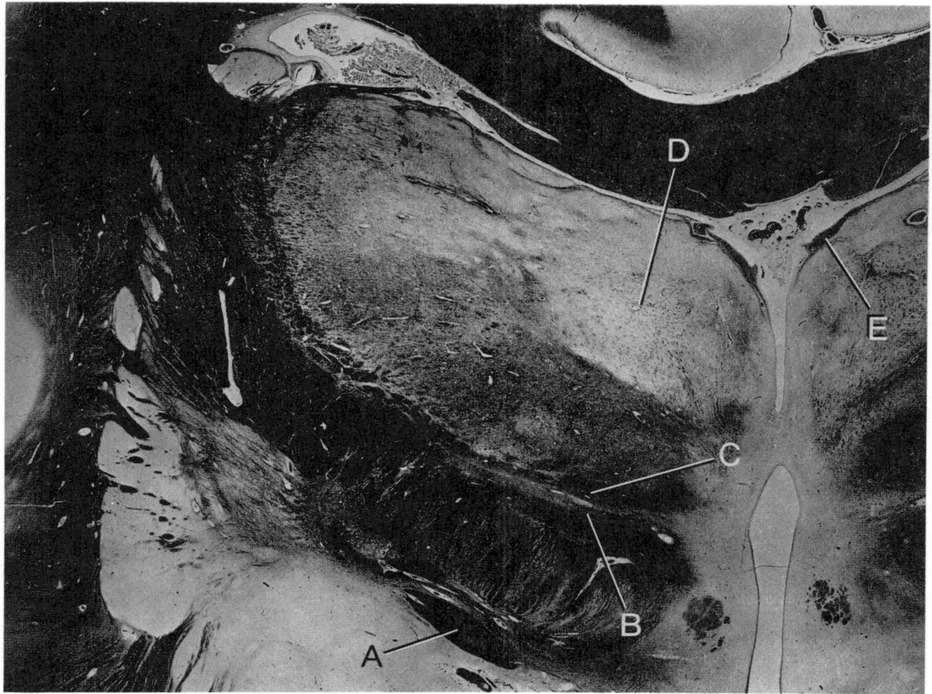

Figure 7.6. Photomicrograph of part of a transverse section through the diencephalon and corpus striatum. (From H. A. Riley, *Atlas of the Basal Ganglia, Brain Stem and Spinal Cord*, 1943; courtesy of Williams & Wilkins, Baltimore.)

7.47. Cells would undergo degeneration following a frontal lobotomy

7.48. Fibers project to habenular nuclei

7.49. Contains pallidofugal fibers and projections from contralateral deep cerebellar nuclei

7.50. Thalamic fasciculus

For each numbered item, select the lettered structure most closely associated with it in Fig. 7.7. Each letter may be selected once, more than once, or not at all.

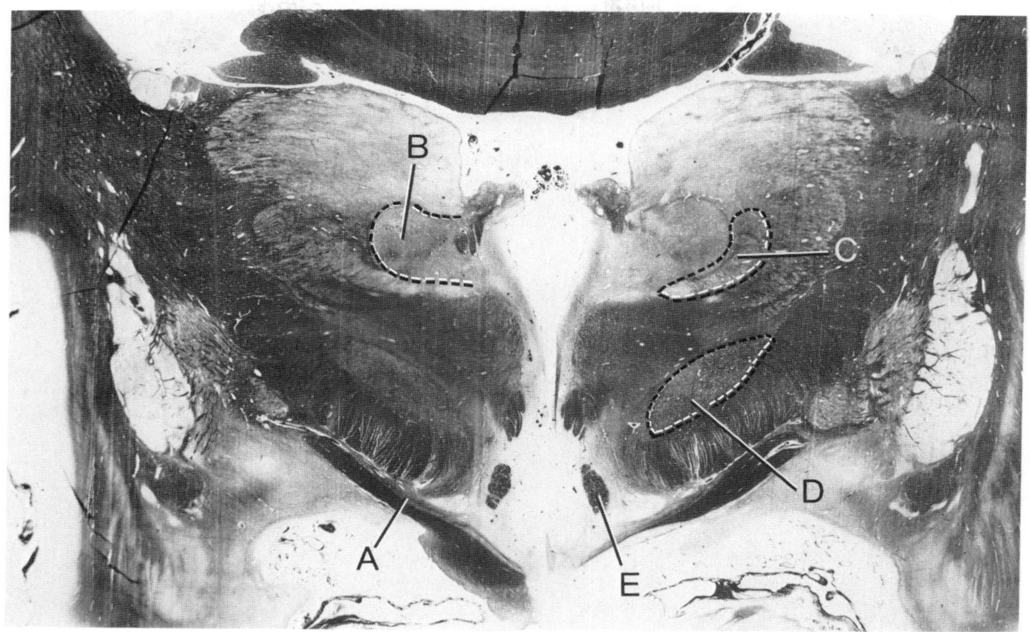

Figure 7.7. Transverse section of the diencephalon and corpus striatum cut perpendicular to the axis of the brain stem. (From H. A. Riley, *Atlas of the Basal Ganglia, Brain Stem and Spinal Cord*, 1943; courtesy of Williams & Wilkins, Baltimore.)

7.51. Derivative of the ventral thalamus

7.52. Largest discrete afferent bundle projecting to hypothalamus

7.53. Receives massive projections from motor cortex

7.54. Afferent input derived from head, face, and intraoral receptors

For each numbered item, select the lettered structure most closely associated with it in Fig. 7.8. Each letter may be selected once, more than once, or not at all.

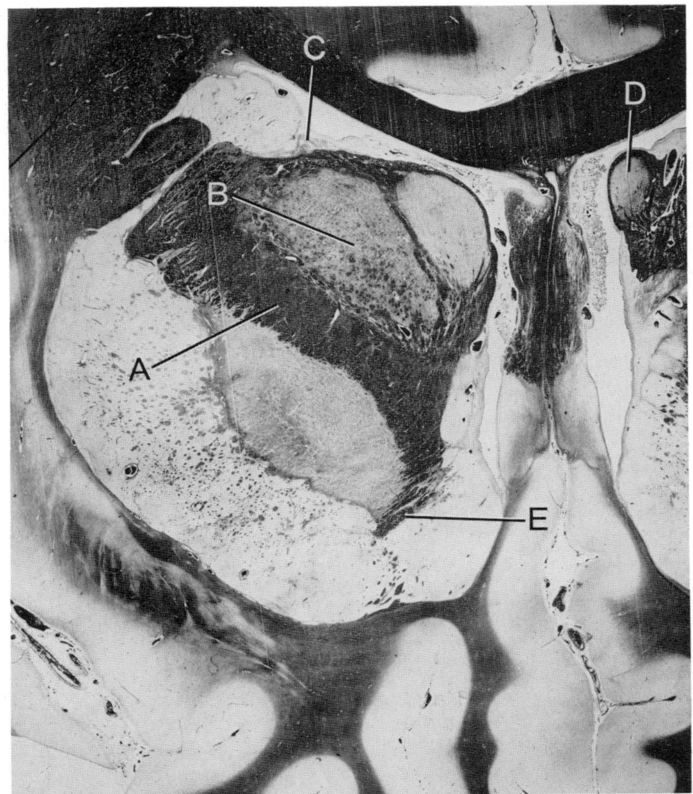

Figure 7.8. Transverse section of the rostral diencephalon and corpus striatum cut perpendicular to the axis of the brain stem. (From H. A. Riley, *Atlas of the Basal Ganglia, Brain Stem and Spinal Cord*, 1943; courtesy of Williams & Wilkins, Baltimore.)

7.55. Anterior tubercle of thalamus

7.56. Contains corticofugal and corticopedal fibers

7.57. Receives input from medial pallidal segment

7.58. Fibers course with a prominent vein and arise from the corticomedial amygdaloid nucleus

For each numbered item, select the lettered structure most closely associated with it in Fig. 7.9. Each letter may be selected once, more than once, or not at all.

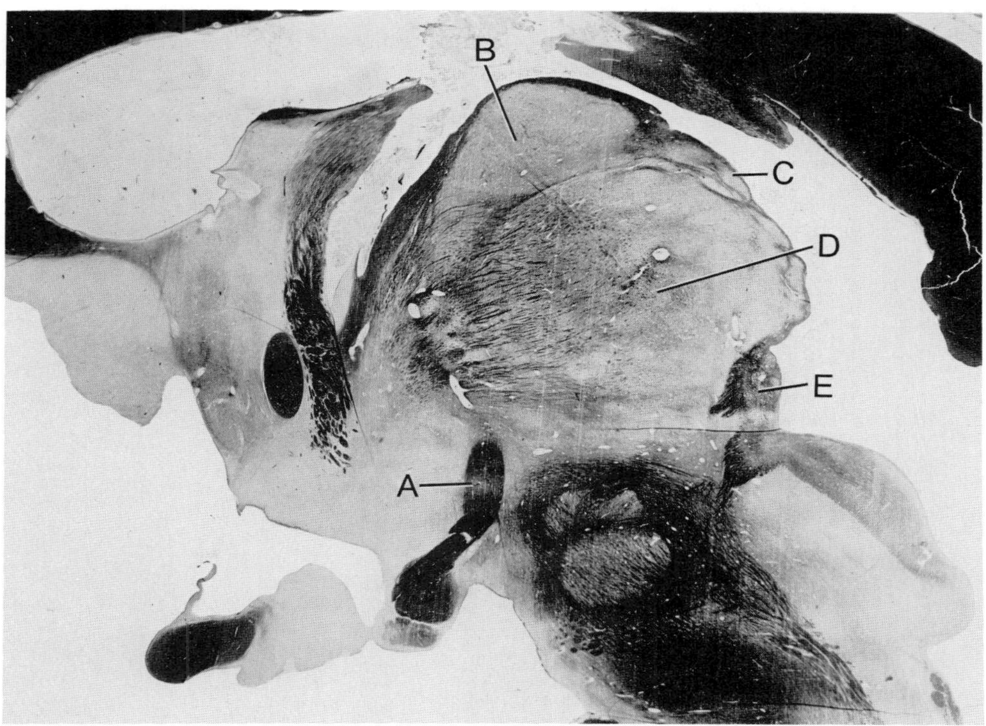

Figure 7.9. Sagittal section of the brain stem close to the midline. (From H. A. Riley, *Atlas of the Basal Ganglia, Brain Stem and Spinal Cord*, 1943; courtesy of Williams & Wilkins, Baltimore.)

7.59. Projects to anterior thalamic nuclei

7.60. Part of the epithalamus

7.61. Large association nucleus of thalamus related to frontal lobe

7.62. Projects fibers to supralimbic cortex of parietal lobe

For each numbered item, select the lettered structure most closely associated with it in Fig. 7.10. Each letter may be selected once, more than once, or not at all.

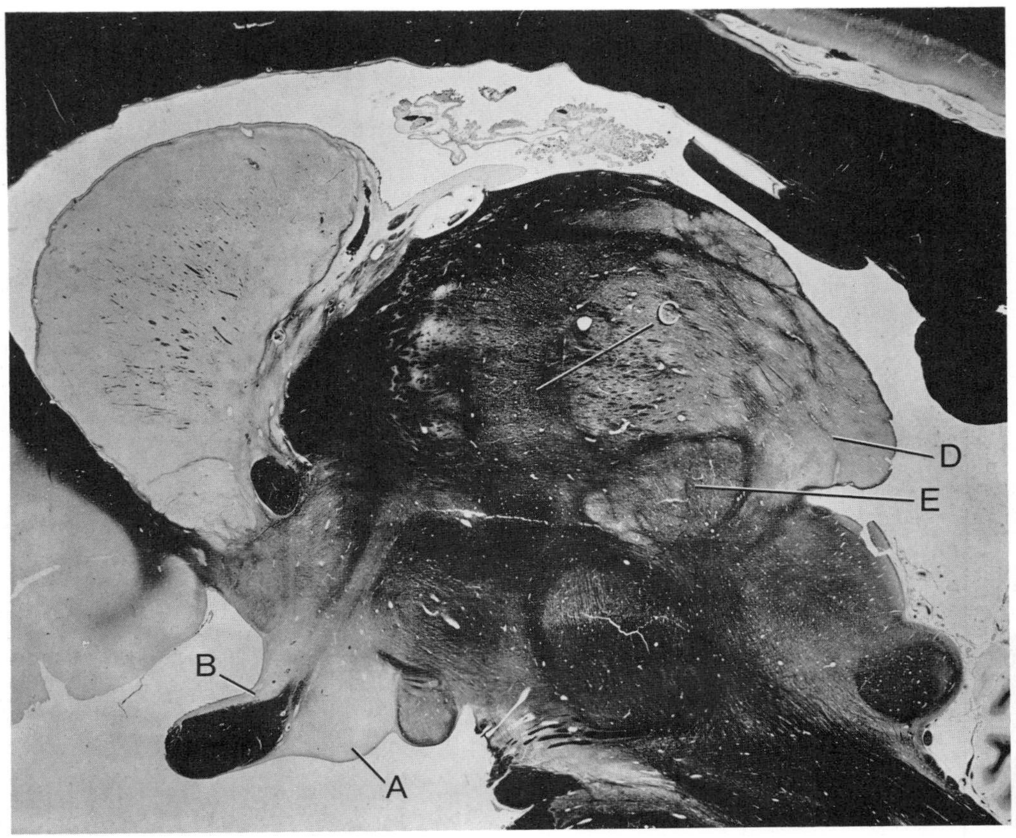

Figure 7.10. Sagittal section of the brain stem lateral to the midline. (From H. A. Riley, *Atlas of the Basal Ganglia, Brain Stem and Spinal Cord*, 1943; courtesy of Williams & Wilkins, Baltimore.)

7.63. Project fibers to the neostriatum

7.64. Ventral tier thalamic nucleus

7.65. Lateral tuberal nuclei

7.66. Projects to neurohypophysis

For each numbered item, select the lettered structure in Fig. 7.11 most closely associated with it. Each letter may be selected once, more than once, or not at all.

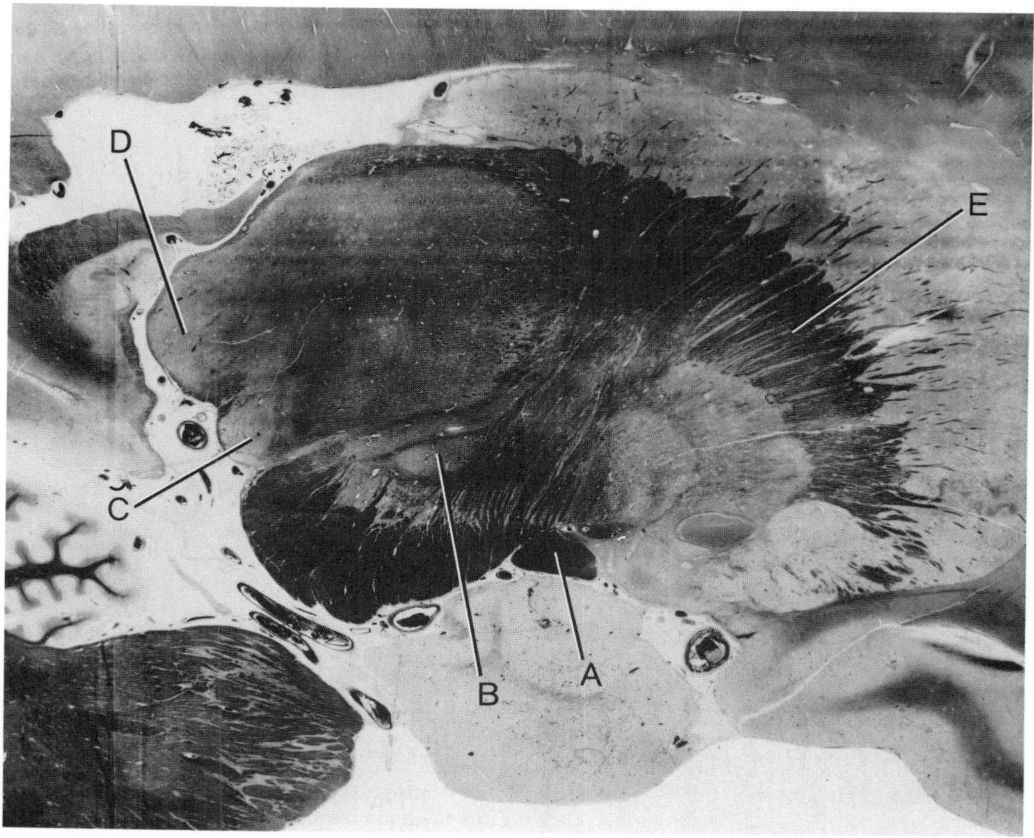

Figure 7.11. Photomicrograph of a sagittal section through lateral parts of the diencephalon and corpus striatum. (From H. A. Riley, *Atlas of the Basal Ganglia, Brain Stem and Spinal Cord*, 1943; courtesy of Williams & Wilkins, Baltimore.)

7.67. Largest thalamic association nucleus

7.68. Contains anterior thalamic radiation

7.69. Projects fibers to all laminae of the lateral geniculate body

7.70. Projects fibers to cortex via the inferior thalamic peduncle

For each numbered item, indicate whether it is associated with

A only (A)
B only (B)
Both A and B (C)
Neither A or B (D)

Questions 7.71–7.74

(A) Ventral posterior thalamic nucleus
(B) Posterior thalamic nucleus
(C) Both
(D) Neither

7.71. Receives input from the primary (S I) somatosensory cortex

7.72. Receives terminals of spinothalamic fibers

7.73. Receives inputs uniquely related to painful and noxious stimuli

7.74. Projects fibers to both the primary (S I) and secondary (SS II) somatosensory cortex

Questions 7.75–7.78

(A) Ventral tier thalamic nuclei
(B) Dorsal tier thalamic nuclei
(C) Both
(D) Neither

7.75. Pulvinar, lateral posterior, and dorsolateral nuclei

7.76. Project profusely to cortex on both banks of the central sulcus

7.77. Intralaminar nuclei

7.78. Corticopedal projections in the posterior limb of the internal capsule

For each numbered item in Fig. 7.12 (*A* and *B* represent lesions), indicate whether it is associated with

A only (A)
B only (B)
Both A and B (C)
Neither A nor B (D)

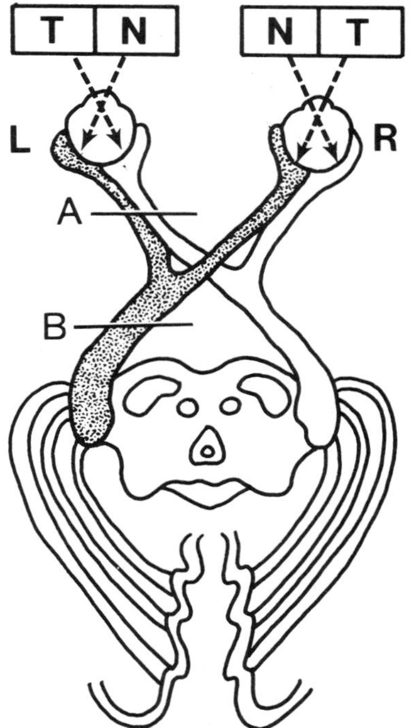

Figure 7.12. Schematic diagram of the visual pathways with lesions indicated at *A* and *B*. *T* and *N* refer to temporal and nasal halves of the retina and *L* and *R* indicate left and right. (From M. B. Carpenter, *Core Text of Neuroanatomy*, 1985; courtesy of Williams & Wilkins, Baltimore.)

7.79. Would *not* abolish direct or consensual pupillary light reflexes to light directed upon the left nasal retina

7.80. Would produce a left homonymous hemianopsia

7.81. Would in time produce transneuronal degeneration in three layers of each lateral geniculate body

7.82. Would produce anisocoria (unequal pupils)

For each of the incomplete statements below, *one* or *more* of the completions given is correct. Choose answer:

(A) Only **1, 2,** and **3** are correct
(B) Only **1** and **3** are correct
(C) Only **2** and **4** are correct
(D) Only **4** is correct
(E) **All** are correct

7.83. The ventral posterior lateral nucleus (pars caudalis) of the thalamus:
(1) receives most impulses concerned with pain
(2) relays impulses concerned with kinesthetic sense and tactile sense to the postcentral gyrus
(3) receives the medial lemniscus and the secondary trigeminal tracts
(4) is somatotopically organized

7.84. Primary retinal afferents from one eye project to:
(1) parts of both lateral geniculate bodies
(2) predominantly to the contralateral superior colliculus
(3) both suprachiasmatic nuclei
(4) the pretectal olivary nuclei

7.85. The intralaminar thalamic nuclei receive inputs from:
(1) globus pallidus
(2) cerebral cortex
(3) central tegmental tract
(4) inferior olivary complex

7.86. Repetitive stimulation of the intralaminar thalamic nuclei at rates of 6–12 per second:
(1) gives rise to an electroencephalographic (EEG) arousal response
(2) produces a recruiting response
(3) can block an on-going recruiting response
(4) results in depolarization and hyperpolarization of cortical dendrites which wax and wane

7.87. In the medial geniculate body:
(1) all subdivisions project to the primary auditory cortex
(2) the dorsal and medial nuclear subdivisions project to a cortical belt surrounding the primary auditory area
(3) the ventral laminated part of the medial geniculate body receives input only from the pericentral nucleus of the inferior colliculus
(4) the ventral laminated nucleus projects to the primary auditory cortex

7.88. The habenular nuclei:
(1) receive inputs from the septal nuclei
(2) receive projections from the medial pallidal segment
(3) project via the fasciculus retroflexus to the interpeduncular nucleus
(4) together with the striae medullares of the thalamus and pineal body, constitute the epithalamus

7.89. The intralaminar thalamic nuclei:
(1) receive major inputs from the brain stem reticular formation, the deep cerebellar nuclei and the cerebral cortex
(2) undergo chromatolytic cell changes following large cortical ablations
(3) project fibers to the neostriatum and to broad areas of the cerebral cortex
(4) project to cerebral cortex only via collaterals of thalamostriate fibers

7.90. The dorsomedial or mediodorsal nucleus of the thalamus:
(1) has been divided into three cytologically distinct parts
(2) has a magnocellular part which receives projections from the amygdaloid nuclear complex
(3) has a paralaminar part with reciprocal connections to the frontal eye field (area 8)
(4) has a parvicellular part that degenerates after frontal lobotomy

7.91. The anterior nuclear group of the thalamus:
(1) receives direct projections from the fornix
(2) receives projections from the hypothalamus
(3) projects to the cingulate cortex
(4) constitutes a link in the "Papez circuit" for emotional expression

7.92. The ventral lateral nucleus of the thalamus:

(1) has three major divisions, pars oralis (VLo), pars caudalis (VLc), and pars medialis (VLm)
(2) has reciprocal connections with the primary somesthetic cortex
(3) projects via VLo to the premotor cortex
(4) receives crossed inputs to VLo and VLm from the deep cerebellar nuclei

7.93. Amacrine cells in the retina:

(1) have no axons
(2) make synaptic contacts with both rods and cones
(3) make synaptic contacts with bipolar and ganglion cells
(4) make no synaptic contacts with other amacrine cells

7.94. Thalamic nuclei, whose stimulation initiates synchronization of electrocortical rhythms, include:

(1) ventral posterolateral (VPLo)
(2) intralaminar
(3) ventral lateral (VLo)
(4) ventral anterior (VApc)

7.95. In the lateral geniculate body:

(1) the monocular crescent of the visual field is represented by the bilaminar segment
(2) binocular fusion occurs
(3) the blind spot is represented by discontinuities in laminae 4 and 6
(4) all laminae project to the striate cortex via the optic radiations

7.96. The ventral posterior thalamic nucleus:

(1) consists of two major portions, ventral posterolateral (VPL) and ventral posteromedial (VPM)
(2) has a caudal part, the ventral posterolateral nucleus (VPLc), which receives fibers of the medial lemniscus and the spinothalamic tract
(3) has a medial part, the ventral posteromedial nucleus (VPM), which receives crossed and uncrossed trigeminothalamic fibers
(4) has a small-celled medial part (VPMpc), which receives uncrossed gustatory projections

7.97. The ventral anterior nucleus (VA) of the thalamus:

(1) consists of two distinct cytological subdivisions
(2) receives projections from the pars reticulata of the substantia nigra in the magnocellular (VAmc) subdivision
(3) receives pallidal projections in the pars principalis (VApc)
(4) projects to all parts of the frontal lobe

7.98. Neurons in the ventral posterolateral nucleus (VPL) of the thalamus:

(1) project ipsilaterally to cortical areas SS I and SS II
(2) are concerned primarily with the perception of tactile and kinesthetic sense
(3) are related to a restricted unchanging receptive field on the contralateral side of the body
(4) receive all thalamic terminations of the spinothalamic tract

7.99. Melatonin in the pineal gland:

(1) is reduced by exposure to light
(2) is synthesized from serotonin
(3) fluctuates in response to the daily cycle of photic input
(4) is regulated by cells of the suprachiasmatic nucleus which control essential enzymes

7.100. In the lateral geniculate body:

(1) the horizontal meridian of the visual field corresponds to an oblique plane that divides the nucleus into medial and lateral segments
(2) the macular region is represented rostrally
(3) central vision is represented caudally on both sides of the horizontal meridian
(4) the monocular crescent of the visual field is represented along the caudal margin

Answers and Explanations*

7.1. **B** Although homonymous visual field defects occur with all lesions of the visual pathways caudal to the optic chiasm, congruent field defects are most common with lesions of the striate cortex. See pp. 259 and 363

7.2. **C** See pp. 259 and 363

7.3. **D** In right geniculate body in layers 1, 4, and 6 and in the 2, 3, and 5 layers of the right lateral geniculate body. See pp. 247 and 249

7.4. **C** See Fig. 9-25

7.5. **C** All cells in the bilaminar segment of the lateral geniculate body, the fused lateral parts of laminae 4 and 6, receive crossed fibers. Cells in lamina I also receive crossed retinal inputs

7.6. **B** The ventral nucleus of the lateral geniculate body has only subcortical projections. The entire lateral geniculate body is a derivative of the ventral thalamus

7.7. **D** Melatonin is produced during periods of darkness. See p. 225

7.8. **A** The inhibitory surround has an amacrine cell interposed between bipolar and ganglion cells. See p. 259

7.9. **B** The medial and lateral geniculate bodies lie lateral and posterior to the internal capsule

7.10. **C** The largest intralaminar thalamic nuclei receive the major projections from the cerebral cortex. See pp. 233–234

7.11. **B** See pp. 253–254

7.12. **E**

7.13. **D**

7.14. **A**

7.15. **B**

7.16. **E** Taste fibers from the nucleus solitarius are uncrossed

7.17. **C** Sensation from most of the cranial dura is transmitted via the trigeminal nerve

7.18. **D** See p. 241

7.19. **C** Inferior pulvinar

7.20. **B** Medial geniculate body

7.21. **A** Cells of the pars reticulata of the substantia nigra

7.22. **D** Lateral geniculate body

7.23. **E** See pp. 238 and 373

7.24. **D** See p. 243

7.25. **B** See p. 239

7.26. **A** See p. 231

7.27. **B** Lesion of optic radiation

7.28. **C** Lesion posterior limb of internal capsule

7.29. **A** Lesion at genu of the internal capsule

7.30. **E** Thalamic lesion

7.31. **E** Zona incerta

7.32. **D** Ventral posterolateral nucleus

7.33. **A** Hypothalamic sulcus

7.34. **B** Prerubral field

7.35. **C** See p. 263

7.36. **A** See p. 261

7.37. **B** The anterior nuclear group are included in this group because of relays from mammillary nuclei and hippocampal formation

7.38. **D** Intralaminar thalamic nuclei project to striatum and diffuse regions of the cortex

7.39. **E**

7.40. **A** An ipsilateral (left) light stimulus would not produce a direct or consensual pupillary response

7.41. **C** Transneuronal degeneration would occur bilaterally in laminae 1, 4, and 6

* All page numbers and illustration citations refer to Carpenter: CORE TEXT OF NEUROANATOMY, 3rd edition; © 1985, Williams & Wilkins.

7.42. **E** A lesion in the striate cortex would produce retrograde cell changes in the parvicellular layers of the ipsilateral lateral geniculate body

7.43. **E** Reticular nucleus of thalamus. See p. 251

7.44. **D** Ventral lateral nucleus of thalamus (VLo)

7.45. **B** Lateral dorsal nucleus

7.46. **C** Mammillothalamic tract

7.47. **D** Dorsomedial nucleus of thalamus

7.48. **E** Stria medullaris

7.49. **C** Thalamic fasciculus

7.50. **C**

7.51. **D** Subthalamic nucleus

7.52. **E** Fornix

7.53. **B** Centromedian nucleus

7.54. **C** Ventral posteromedial nucleus (VPM)

7.55. **D**

7.56. **A** Posterior limb of internal capsule

7.57. **B** Ventral anterior thalamic nucleus (VApc)

7.58. **C** Stria terminalis

7.59. **A** Mammillothalamic tract

7.60. **E** Habenular nuclei

7.61. **D** Dorsomedial nucleus

7.62. **C** Lateral dorsal nucleus. See p. 237

7.63. **E** Centromedian nucleus

7.64. **C** Ventral lateral nucleus

7.65. **A** Lateral tuberal nuclei of hypothalamus

7.66. **B** Supraoptic nucleus of hypothalamus

7.67. **D** Pulvinar

7.68. **E** Anterior limb of internal capsule

7.69. **A** Optic tract

7.70. **C** Medial geniculate body. See p. 255

7.71. **A** Corticothalamic projections from S I pass to the ventrobasal complex, but not to the posterior thalamic nucleus. See p. 386

7.72. **C** See pp. 241 and 243

7.73. **D** Neither is uniquely related to pain

7.74. **A** See p. 243

7.75. **B** Nuclei in the dorsal part of the lateral nuclear group, known as the dorsal tier thalamic nuclei, are best developed in caudal regions of the thalamus

7.76. **A** Ventral tier thalamic nuclei include VA, VL, and VP

7.77. **D**

7.78. **C** Both groups of thalamic nuclei project fibers to the cerebral cortex via the posterior limb of the internal capsule

7.79. **B**

7.80. **D**

7.81. **A** Transneuronal degeneration would occur in layers 1, 4, and 6 on the right and in layers 2, 3, and 5 on the left

7.82. **D**

7.83. **C** VPLc receives the medial lemniscus and spinothalamic tracts, is somatotopically organized and projects to the postcentral gyrus

7.84. **E** See pp. 257–258

7.85. **A** See pp. 233–235

7.86. **C** See pp. 264 and 353

7.87. **C** See pp. 245–246 and 374–375

7.88. **E** See p. 223

7.89. **B** Some cells in the central lateral and paracentral thalamic nuclei receive input from the midbrain reticular formation and project directly to the cerebral cortex. See p. 236

7.90. **E** See pp. 230–231

7.91. **E** See pp. 229 and 338

7.92. **B** See pp. 240 and 384

7.93. **B** See p. 255

7.94. **C** See pp. 239 and 264

7.95. **B** See p. 247

7.96. **E** See pp. 241–243

7.97. **A** VA projects to frontal cortex rostral to the precentral gyrus. See p. 239

7.98. **A** Some fibers of the spinothalamic tract terminate in the posterior thalamic nucleus

7.99. **E** See p. 225

7.100. **B** See p. 249

8

Hypothalamus

Questions

Select the one best answer

8.1. Hyperphagia, obesity, and ferocious behavior in animals may result from:

(A) lesions in the anterior hypothalamus
(B) bilateral lesions of the corticomedial amygdala
(C) lesions in the lateral hypothalamic nuclei
(D) bilateral lesions in the ventromedial hypothalamic nuclei
(E) extensive decortications

8.2. A young boy with a bitemporal hemianopsia, persistant hyperpyrexia (high temperature), diabetes insipidus, and increased intracranial pressure most likely has:

(A) a pituitary adenoma
(B) destruction of the neural lobe of the hypophysis
(C) a tumor of the optic nerve
(D) an expanding lesion involving the anterior hypothalamus
(E) a lesion of the supraopticohypophysial tract

8.3. Afferent input to the hypothalamus is derived principally from:

(A) the hippocampal formation, amygdaloid nuclear complex, and the septal nuclei
(B) anterior, medial, and periventricular thalamic nuclei
(C) the midbrain reticular formation
(D) direct cortical projections
(E) mammillary peduncle

8.4. The magnocellular supraoptic and paraventricular nuclei are concerned with:

(A) the elaboration of hormone releasing factors
(B) temperature regulation
(C) water and food intake
(D) the antidiuretic hormone and oxytocin
(E) mechanisms that regulate sleep

8.5. A hypothalamic lesion associated with complete loss of thermoregulatory control (i.e., poikilothermia) is most likely located in:

(A) the anterior hypothalamus
(B) the lateral hypothalamus
(C) the posterior hypothalamus
(D) the mammillary nuclei
(E) the medial forebrain bundle

8.6. The neuronal pacemaker (biological clock) entrained by photic cues is:

(A) hypothalamic paraventricular nucleus
(B) lateral geniculate body pars ventralis
(C) lateral geniculate body pars dorsalis
(D) suprachiasmatic nuclei
(E) supraoptic nucleus

8.7. The hypothalamus is concerned with each of the following, *except*:

(A) water balance
(B) control of blood pressure
(C) physiological correlates of emotion
(D) control of endocrine functions
(E) appetite

8.8. Electrical stimulation of the hypothalamus in unanesthetized animals can produce all of the following, *except*:
(A) pseudo-affective rage
(B) enormous "thirst"
(C) ovulation
(D) release of gonadotropic hormone
(E) changes in body temperature

8.9. Hypothalamically induced rage reactions can be blocked by:
(A) cortical lesions
(B) midbrain lesions
(C) lesions in amygdala
(D) lesions in the adenohypophysis
(E) bilateral lesions in the ventromedial hypothalamic nucleus

8.10. Prolactin secretions of the anterior pituitary can be reduced by:
(A) β-endorphins
(B) dopamine agonists (e.g., bromocriptine)
(C) serotonin
(D) norepinephrine
(E) oxytocin

For each numbered item, select the one heading most closely associated with it. Each lettered heading may be selected once, more than once, or not at all.

Questions 8.11–8.14

(A) Dopamine
(B) Noradrenergic axons
(C) β-Endorphin
(D) Vasopressin
(E) Enkephalin

8.11. Natural occurring peptide in intermediate lobe and adenohypophysis

8.12. Cells of arcuate nucleus

8.13. Medial forebrain bundle

8.14. Distinctive cells in paraventricular and supraoptic nuclei

Questions 8.15–8.18

(A) Circadian rhythms
(B) Magnocellular hypothalamic nuclei
(C) Sexually dimorphic nuclei
(D) Median eminence
(E) Tuberal nuclei

8.15. Preoptic region

8.16. Suprachiasmatic nuclei

8.17. Arcuate nuclei

8.18. Lateral hypothalamus

Questions 8.19–8.22

(A) Satiety center
(B) Feeding center
(C) Diabetes insipidus
(D) Hyperpyrexia (abnormal high body temperature)
(E) Poikilothermia

8.19. Bilateral lesions in rostral hypothalamus

8.20. Bilateral lesions in posterior hypothalamus

8.21. Lateral hypothalamic nuclei

8.22. Lesions in this site are associated with ferocious behavior, obesity, and hyperphagia

For each numbered item, select the one lettered structure most closely associated with it in Fig. 8.1. Each lettered heading may be selected once, more than once, or not at all.

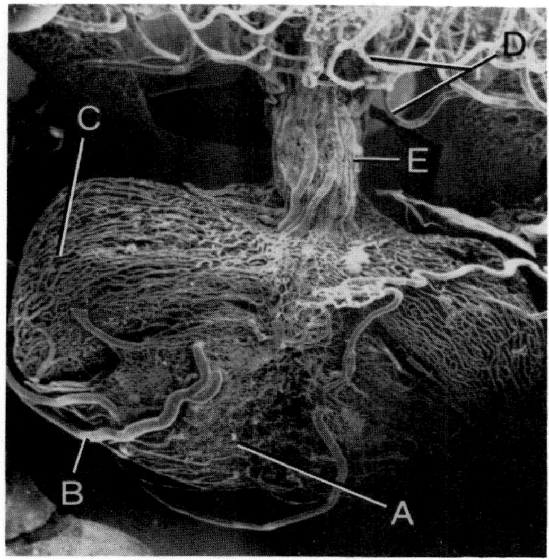

Figure 8.1. Scanning electron micrograph of vascular casts of the hypophysis, infundibulum, and median eminence in a monkey.

8.23. Hypophysial portal vessels

8.24. Site of action of hypophysiotrophic neuropeptides

8.25. Contains terminals of hypothalamic neurosecretory fibers

8.26. Superior hypophysial arteries

For each numbered item, select the one heading most closely associated with it in Fig. 8.2. Each lettered heading may be selected once, more than once, or not at all.

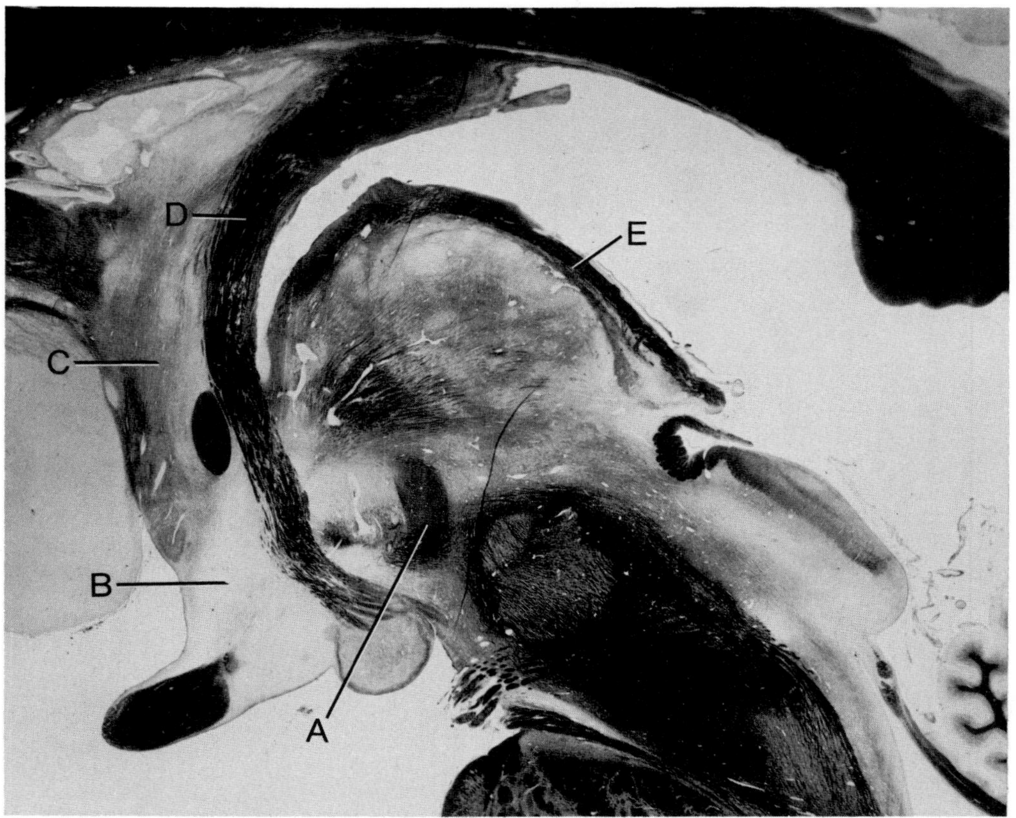

Figure 8.2. Sagittal section of the human brain stem near the midline (Weigert's myelin stain).

8.27. Septal region

8.28. Preoptic area

8.29. Projects fibers to thalamus and midbrain tegmentum

8.30. Distributes fibers to septal nuclei, lateral preoptic area, hypothalamus, and to the anterior and rostral intralaminar thalamic nuclei

For each numbered item, indicate whether it is associated in Fig. 8.3 with

A only (A)
B only (B)
Both A and B (C)
Neither A nor B (D)

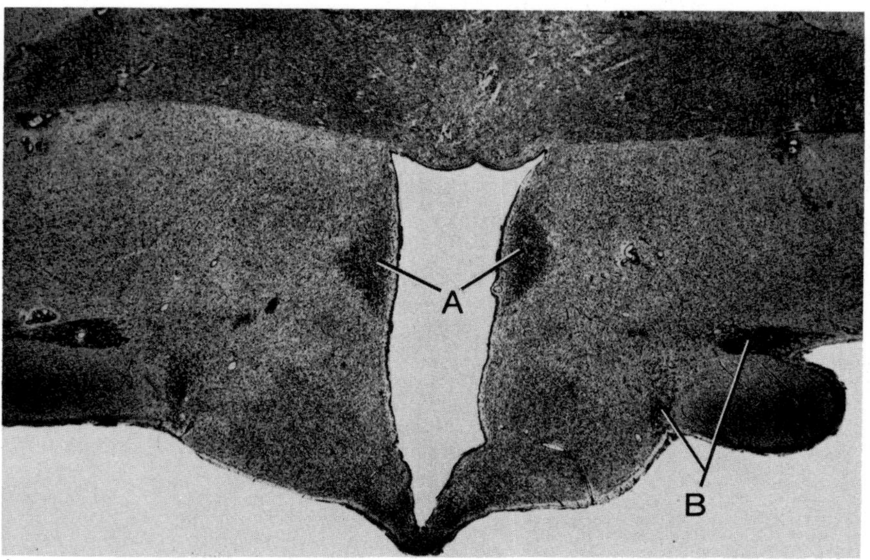

Figure 8.3. Photomicrograph of a transverse section of the human diencephalon at the level of the anterior commissure (cresyl violet stain).

8.31. Vasopressin and oxytocin

8.32. Projects fibers to thoracic, lumbar, and sacral spinal levels

8.33. Peptide hormones are conjugated with neurophysin

8.34. Fibers project to adenohypophysis

For each numbered item, indicate whether it is associated with

A only (A)
B only (B)
Both A and B (C)
Neither A or B (D)

Questions 8.35–8.38

(A) Paraventricular nuclei
(B) Supraoptic nuclei
(C) Both
(D) Neither

8.35. Parvicellular elements project to spinal cord and vagal nuclei

8.36. Cells secrete vasopressin

8.37. Magnocellular elements project to neurohypophysis

8.38. Neurosecretion transported by hypophysial portal system

Questions 8.39–8.42

(A) Medial parabrachial nuclei
(B) Lateral parabrachial nuclei
(C) Both
(D) Neither

8.39. Receive special visceral afferent (SVA) input

8.40. Project to medial preoptic region, paraventricular, dorsomedial, and lateral nuclei of hypothalamus

8.41. Receive general visceral afferent (GVA) input from solitary nuclear complex

8.42. Involved in consumatory behavior

Questions 8.43–8.46

(A) Medial hypothalamic nuclei
(B) Lateral hypothalamus
(C) Both
(D) Neither

8.43. Input from amygdaloid complex

8.44. Input from hippocampal formation and subiculum

8.45. Contains ascending and descending fibers in medial forebrain bundle

8.46. Contains neurosecretory nuclei that produce releasing hormones

For each of the incomplete statements below, *one* or *more* of the completions given is correct. Choose answer:

(A) Only **1, 2,** and **3** are correct
(B) Only **1** and **3** are correct
(C) Only **2** and **4** are correct
(D) Only **4** is correct
(E) **All** are correct

8.47. The anterior and medial hypothalamic areas:
(1) contain a satiety center
(2) are concerned with parasympathetic responses
(3) influence copulatory behavior
(4) receive afferents from the corticomedial amygdala

8.48. The medial forebrain bundle:
(1) is a multineuronal, multisynaptic pathway
(2) traverses the lateral hypothalamus nucleus
(3) extends from septal nuclei to midbrain
(4) represents largely an efferent system

8.49. The arcuate nucleus of the hypothalamus:
(1) is involved in feeding behavior
(2) secretes hormonal releasing factors
(3) sends axons to the posterior pituitary
(4) releases secretion into the hypophysial portal system

8.50. Hypothalamic area(s) related to ovulation is(are) the:
(1) mammillary body
(2) lateral nucleus
(3) paraventricular nucleus
(4) preoptic region

8.51. The hypothalamus:
(1) receives major limbic input via the entorhinal cortex and hippocampal formation
(2) has reciprocal connections with midbrain tegmentum
(3) exerts influences upon cingulate cortex via thalamic nuclei
(4) has reciprocal connections with the amygdala

8.52. The hypothalamus:
(1) extends from the lamina terminalis to the mammillary bodies
(2) is present on both sides of the third ventricle beneath the hypothalamic sulcus
(3) has a median eminence which forms the floor of the third ventricle
(4) is roughly divided into medial and lateral areas by fibers of the fornix

8.53. The median eminence:
(1) represents the anatomical interface between brain and the anterior pituitary
(2) contains tanocytes
(3) forms part of the floor of the third ventricle
(4) is the region rostral to the optic chiasm

8.54. Reciprocal connections exist between hypothalamic nuclei and the:
(1) amygdaloid nuclear complex
(2) midbrain tegmentum
(3) septal nuclei
(4) substantia innominata

8.55. Neurons in the anterior hypothalamus sensitive to increases in blood temperature indirectly cause:
(1) vasodilatation of cutaneous blood vessels
(2) sweating
(3) rapid shallow respiration (in animals)
(4) hyperthermia

8.56. Increases in the osmotic pressure of the blood in the hypothalamus:
(1) increase activity in neurons of the supraoptic and paraventricular nuclei
(2) result in the release of antidiuretic hormone
(3) create "thirst"
(4) causes a depletion of antidiuretic in the neurohypophysis

8.57. Pseudoaffective reactions induced in unanesthetized animals by electrical stimulation:

(1) vary with the site stimulated
(2) are related to stimulus strength
(3) are observed only during stimulation
(4) are goal directed

8.58. In the hypothalamus, dopamine:

(1) is synthesized in cells of the arcuate nucleus
(2) is secreted into hypophysial capillaries
(3) inhibits the release of prolactin from the adenohypophysis
(4) is all converted to norepinephrine

8.59. The suprachiasmatic nucleus, involved in entraining functions relative to melatonin secretion, receives:

(1) a bilateral input from the retina
(2) projections from the pineal
(3) an indirect input from the ventral lateral geniculate nucleus
(4) fibers from the superior colliculus

8.60. The magnocellular hypothalamic nuclei:

(1) project fibers to the neurohypophysis
(2) are located in the supraoptic region
(3) are the paraventricular and supraoptic nuclei
(4) contain cytoplasmic colloidal inclusions

Answers and Explanations*

8.1. **D** Both lesions and stimulation of the ventromedial hypothalamic nuclei produce ferocious behavior. See p. 287

8.2. **D** See p. 284

8.3. **A** See Figs. 10-9 and 10-11

8.4. **D** See pp. 278–288

8.5. **C** A lesion in the posterior hypothalamus also destroys descending projections from the anterior hypothalamus. See p. 285

8.6. **D** The suprachiasmatic nuclei receive retinohypothalamic inputs

8.7. **B** Blood pressure is controlled by cell groups in the lower brain stem. See p. 126 and Fig. 5-13

8.8. **E** Mechanisms that control body temperature are slow acting

8.9. **B** See p. 288

8.10. **B** See p. 282

8.11. **C** See p. 282

8.12. **A** See p. 282 and Fig. 10-15

8.13. **B** Noradrenergic axons ascend to the hypothalamus from lower brain stem levels. See p. 282

8.14. **D** In the supraoptic and paraventricular nuclei, different cells are associated with oxytocin and vasopressin. See p. 278

8.15. **C** The preoptic region contains sexually dimorphic nuclei

8.16. **A** See pp. 225 and 267

8.17. **D** See pp. 267 and 279 and Fig. 10-15

8.18. **E** The tuberal nuclei lie in the lateral hypothalamus. See Fig. 10-2

8.19. **D** The rostral hypothalamus is concerned with parasympathetic functions essential for heat dissipation

8.20. **E** All thermoregulator mechanisms are destroyed or interrupted

8.21. **B** Lesions in the lateral hypothalamic nuclei abolish feeding desire

8.22. **A** Lesions in the ventromedial hypothalamic nuclei produce ferocious behavior and hyperphagia and this region is called the satiety center

8.23. **E** See Fig. 10-13

8.24. **C** Adenohypophysis

8.25. **A** Neurohypophysis

8.26. **D**

8.27. **C** The septal region is on both sides of the septum pellucidum and lies rostral to the preoptic area

8.28. **B**

8.29. **A** Mammillary princeps divides and projects fibers to thalamus and midbrain. See Figs. 10-6 and 10-8

8.30. **D** Structure is the fornix.

8.31. **C** Magnocellular supraoptic and paraventricular nuclei

8.32. **A** Small cells in paraventricular nuclei project to spinal levels. See Fig. 4-15

8.33. **C**

8.34. **D** Supraoptic and paraventricular nuclei do not project fibers to adenohypophysis

8.35. **A** See p. 95

8.36. **C**

8.37. **C**

8.38. **D**

8.39. **A** Medial parabrachial nuclei receive SVA input from nucleus solitarius. See Fig. 5-21

8.40. **B** See p. 273

8.41. **B** Lateral parabrachial nuclei receive GVA input from nucleus solitarius

8.42. **C** See Fig. 10-9

8.43. **C** See p. 271

* All page numbers and illustration citations refer to Carpenter: CORE TEXT OF NEUROANATOMY, 3rd edition; © 1985, Williams & Wilkins.

8.44. **A** See pp. 271 and 337
8.45. **B** See Figs. 10-8 and 10-11
8.46. **A** See p. 279
8.47. **E**
8.48. **A** See p. 275
8.49. **C** See p. 279
8.50. **D** See p. 286
8.51. **E** See Fig. 10-11
8.52. **E** See Fig. 10-1 and pp. 265–266
8.53. **A** The median eminence lies caudal to the optic chiasm
8.54. **A** The substantia innominata has widespread projections to cortex
8.55. **A** See p. 284
8.56. **E** See p. 285
8.57. **E** See p. 287
8.58. **A** See Fig. 10-15 and p. 282
8.59. **B** See p. 273
8.60. **E** See pp. 267 and 277

9

Corpus Striatum and Related Nuclei

Questions

Select the one best answer

9.1. Embryological derivatives of the striatal ridge in the telencephalic vesicle include the following, *except for*:
(A) head of the caudate nucleus
(B) the amygdala
(C) the putamen
(D) the tail of the caudate nucleus
(E) the globus pallidus

9.2. A form of reciprocal connections exists between:
(A) the subthalamic nucleus and the substantia nigra
(B) the globus pallidus and the substantia nigra
(C) subthalamic nucleus and the medial pallidal segment
(D) neostriatum and the substantia nigra
(E) neostriatum and the centromedian nucleus

9.3. Collaterals of pallidothalamic fibers projecting to the ventral anterior and ventral lateral thalamic nuclei terminate in:
(A) pulvinar
(B) lateral posterior nucleus
(C) anterior nucleus group
(D) dorsal medial nucleus
(E) centromedian nucleus

9.4. Hemiballism occurs contralateral to a lesion in the:
(A) caudate nucleus
(B) subthalamic nucleus
(C) putamen
(D) globus pallidus
(E) substantia nigra

9.5. The major output systems of the corpus striatum and related nuclei arise from:
(A) putamen
(B) pars compacta of substantia nigra
(C) medial pallidal segment and pars reticulata of substantia nigra
(D) lateral pallidal segment
(E) subthalamic nucleus

9.6. One of the following forms of dyskinesia is usually associated with spastic paresis:
(A) chorea
(B) paralysis agitans
(C) hemiballism
(D) athetosis
(E) myoclonus

9.7. The most massive input to the neostriatum arises from the:
(A) substantia nigra
(B) intralaminar thalamic nuclei
(C) cerebral cortex
(D) amygdala
(E) raphe nuclei

9.8. Gamma (γ)-aminobutyric acid (GABA) is considered the predominant neurotransmitter in all of the following, *except*:
(A) strionigral fibers
(B) striopallidal fibers
(C) subthalamopallidal fibers
(D) corticostriate fibers
(E) pallidonigral fibers

9.9. Brains of patients with Huntington's disease (chorea) demonstrate all of the following, *except*:
(A) reduced striatal concentrations of γ-aminobutyric acid (GABA)
(B) reduced striatal choline acetyltransferase (ChAc)
(C) reduced striatal tyrosine hydroxylase (T-OH)
(D) reduced substance P and enkephalin in the globus pallidus
(E) reduced substance P and enkephalin in the substantia nigra

9.10. Pallidothalamic projections:
(A) overlap those originating in the substantia nigra
(B) overlap those originating from the contralateral deep cerebellar nuclei
(C) impinge upon nuclei that project to the primary motor cortex
(D) have synaptic articulations with neurons projecting upon premotor cortex
(E) originate from cells in the lateral pallidal segment

For each numbered item, select the one heading most closely associated with it. Each lettered heading may be selected once, more than once, or not at all.

Questions 9.11–9.14

(A) Substance P
(B) Gamma (γ)-aminobutyric acid
(C) Glutamate
(D) Serotonin
(E) Dopamine

9.11. Inhibitory neurotransmitter transported to both the substantia nigra and putamen

9.12. Excitatory neurotransmitter of corticostriate fibers

9.13. Weak excitatory neurotransmitter acting upon both spiny and aspiny striatal neurons

9.14. Inhibitory neurotransmitter acting upon both segments of globus pallidus and the substantia nigra

Questions 9.15–9.18

(A) Medial pallidal segment
(B) Subthalamic nucleus
(C) Centromedian nucleus
(D) Substantia nigra, pars reticulate
(E) Putamen

9.15. Receives inputs from lateral pallidal segment, motor cortex, and centromedian nucleus

9.16. Projects to thalamic nuclei and the superior colliculus

9.17. Receives collaterals of pallidothalamic projections

9.18. Afferents have serotonin, dopamine, and glutamate as neurotransmitters

For each numbered item, select the lettered structure in Fig. 9.1 most closely associated with it. Each lettered structure may be selected once, more than once, or not at all.

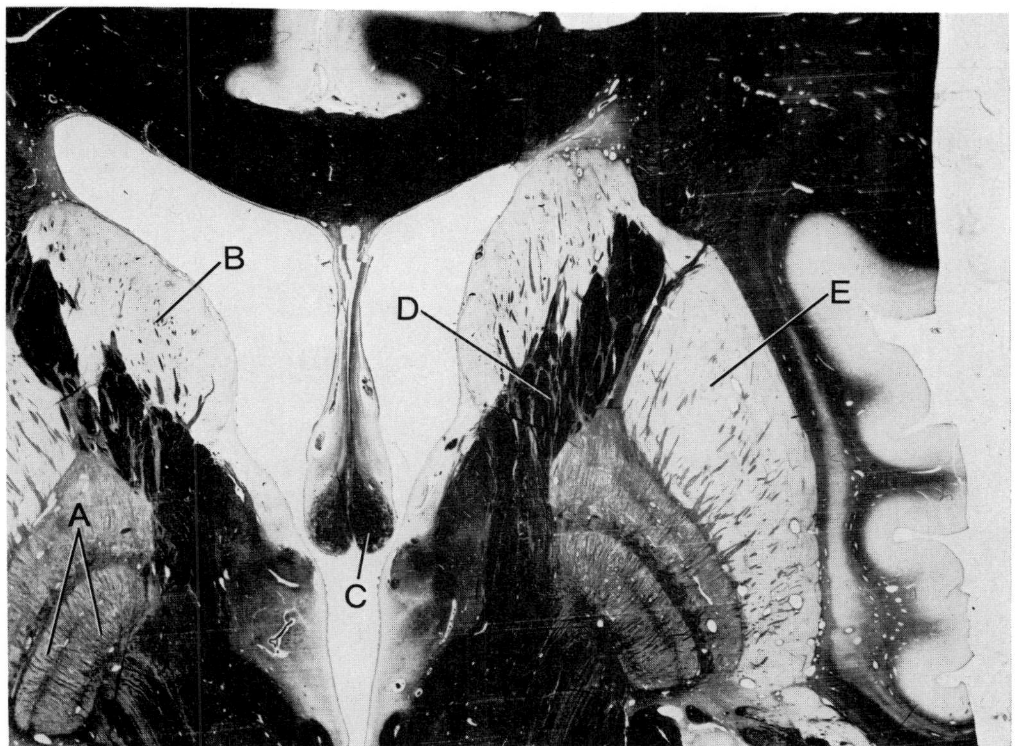

Figure 9.1. Horizontal section through the basal ganglia (Weigert's myelin stain). (From H. A. Riley, *Atlas of the Basal Ganglia, Brain Stem and Spinal Cord*, 1943; courtesy of Williams & Wilkins, Baltimore.)

9.19. Receives bilateral, somatotopical projections from the primary motor cortex, area 4

9.20. Gives rise to the ansa lenticularis and the lenticular fasciculus

9.21 Receives fibers from the ipsilateral prefrontal cortex

9.22. Represents projections from the hippocampal formation and the subiculum

For each numbered item, select the one heading most closely associated with it. Each lettered heading may be selected once, more than once, or not at all.

Questions 9.23–9.26

(A) Serotonin
(B) Dopamine
(C) Gamma (γ)-aminobutyric acid (GABA)
(D) Substance P
(E) L-Dopa

9.23. Passes the blood-brain barrier and is systemically decarboxylated

9.24. Transported to the locus ceruleus, substantia nigra, and striatum

9.25. Excitatory neurotransmitter in forebrain, brain stem, and spinal cord

9.26. Synthesized by type I spiny striatal neurons

For each numbered item, select the lettered structure in Fig. 9.2 most closely associated with it. Each lettered structure may be selected once, more than once, or not at all.

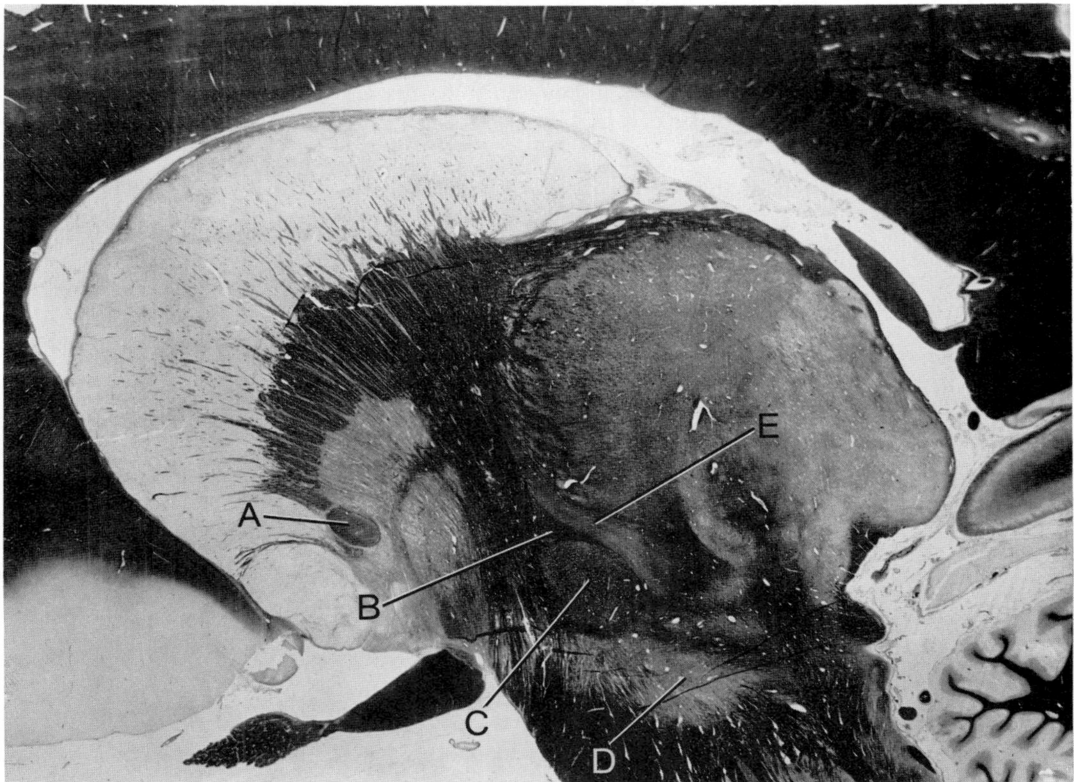

Figure 9.2. Sagittal section through the basal ganglia and diencephalon (Weigert's myelin stain). (From H. A. Riley, *Atlas of the Basal Ganglia, Brain Stem and Spinal Cord*, 1943; courtesy of Williams & Wilkins, Baltimore.)

9.27. Separates the lenticular fasciculus and thalamic fasciculus

9.28. Projects fibers to both the globus pallidus and substantia nigra

9.29. Lenticular fasciculus

9.30. Receives projections of spiny striatal neurons

For each numbered item, select the one heading most closely associated with it. Each lettered heading may be selected once, more than once, or not at all.

Questions 9.31–9.34

(A) Choreoid dyskinesia
(B) Ballism
(C) Tremor at rest
(D) Tremor association with voluntary movement
(E) Athetosis

9.31. Associated with impaired synthesis and transport of dopamine

9.32. May appear in a patient with paralysis agitans if the dopamine levels greatly exceed that of (γ-aminobutyric acid (GABA)

9.33. Associated with lesions of the dentate nucleus

9.34. Results from a lesion that removes inhibitory influences acting upon the globus pallidus

For each numbered item, select the lettered structure most closely associated with it in Fig. 9.3. Each lettered heading may be selected once, more than once, or not at all.

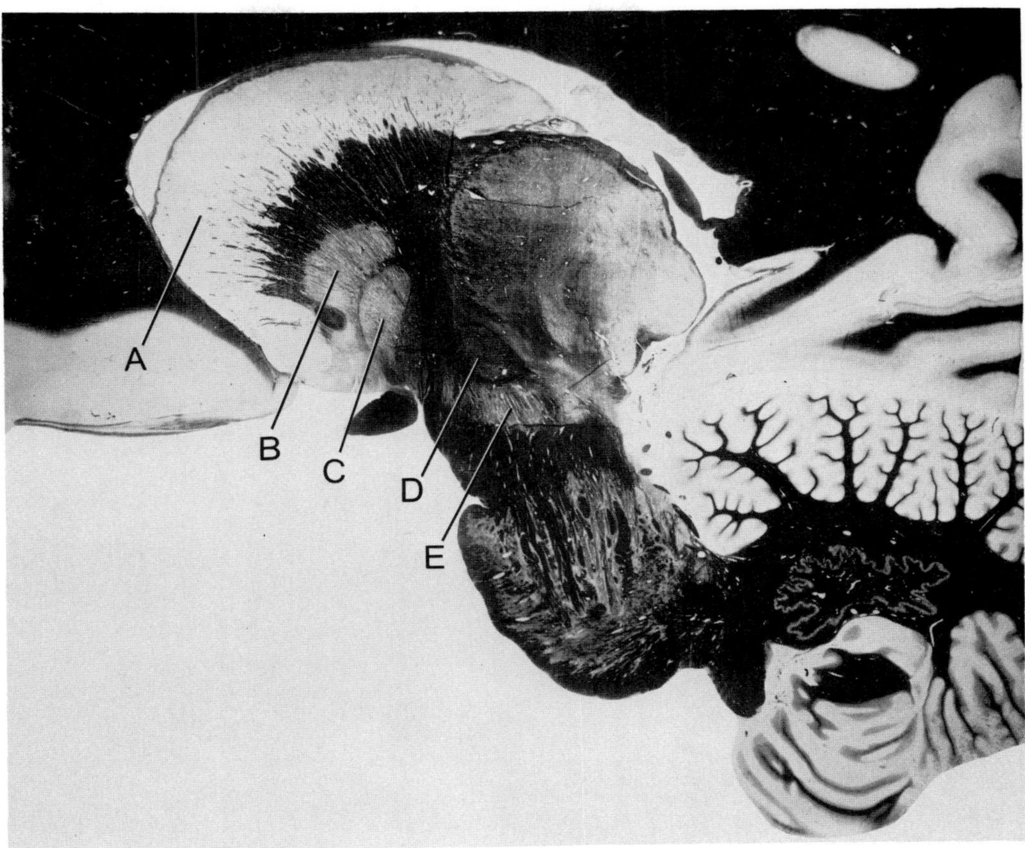

Figure 9.3. Sagittal section through basal ganglia, brain stem and cerebellum (Weigert's myelin stain). (From H. A. Riley, *Atlas of the Basal Ganglia, Brain Stem and Spinal Cord*, 1943; courtesy of Williams & Wilkins, Baltimore.)

9.35. An injection of a γ-aminobutyric acid (GABA) antagonist would produce contralateral ballistic activity

9.36. An injection of kainic acid would diminish GABA in the globus pallidus and substantia nigra

9.37. An injection of horseradish peroxidase (HRP) would retrogradely label neurons in the cerebral cortex, the centromedian nucleus, and in the pars compacta of the substantia nigra

9.38. Immunocytochemical staining would reveal predominantly fibers and terminals containing GABA and enkephalin

9.39. Immunocytochemical staining would reveal fibers containing GABA and substance P

For each numbered item, select the lettered structure most closely associated with it in Fig. 9.4. Each lettered heading may be selected once, more than once, or not at all.

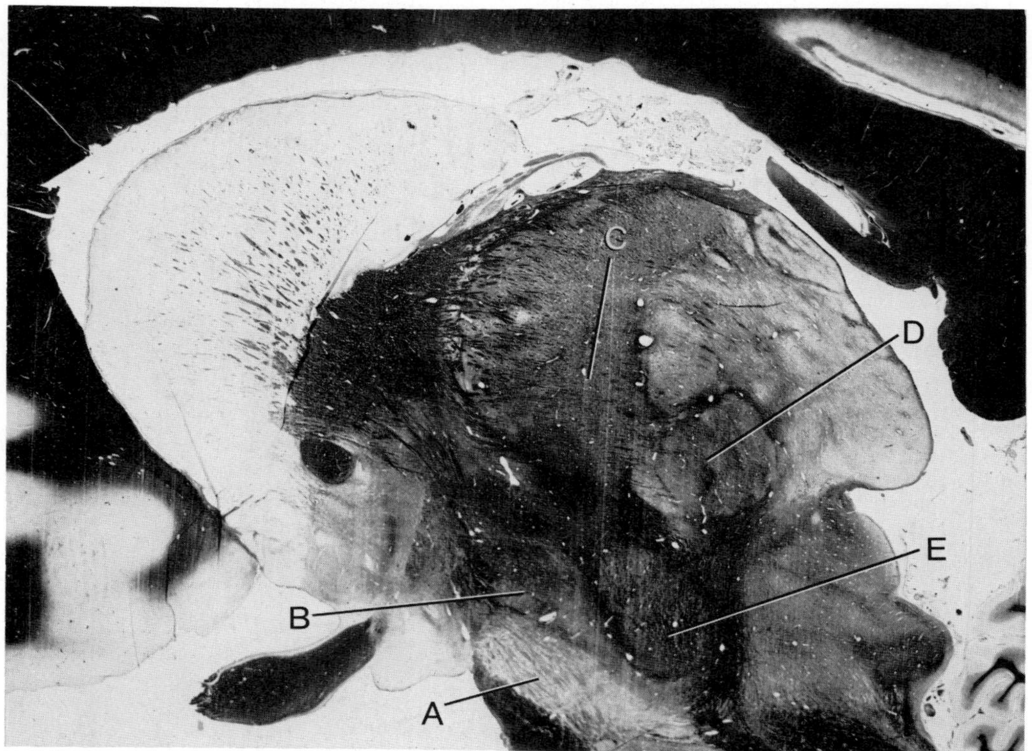

Figure 9.4. Medial sagittal section through caudate nucleus, putamen, and thalamus (Weigert's myelin stain). (From H. A. Riley, *Atlas of the Basal Ganglia, Brain Stem and Spinal Cord*, 1943; courtesy of Williams & Wilkins, Baltimore.)

9.40. Single cells project fibers to both the globus pallidus and the substantia nigra

9.41. Cells project fibers to the neostriatum and broad regions of the cerebral cortex

9.42. Some cells in this structure project to both the thalamus and superior colliculus

9.43. Cells in this nucleus project to brain stem nuclei and spinal cord

For each numbered item, select the lettered structure in Fig. 9.5 most closely associated with it. Each lettered structure may be selected once, more than once, or not at all.

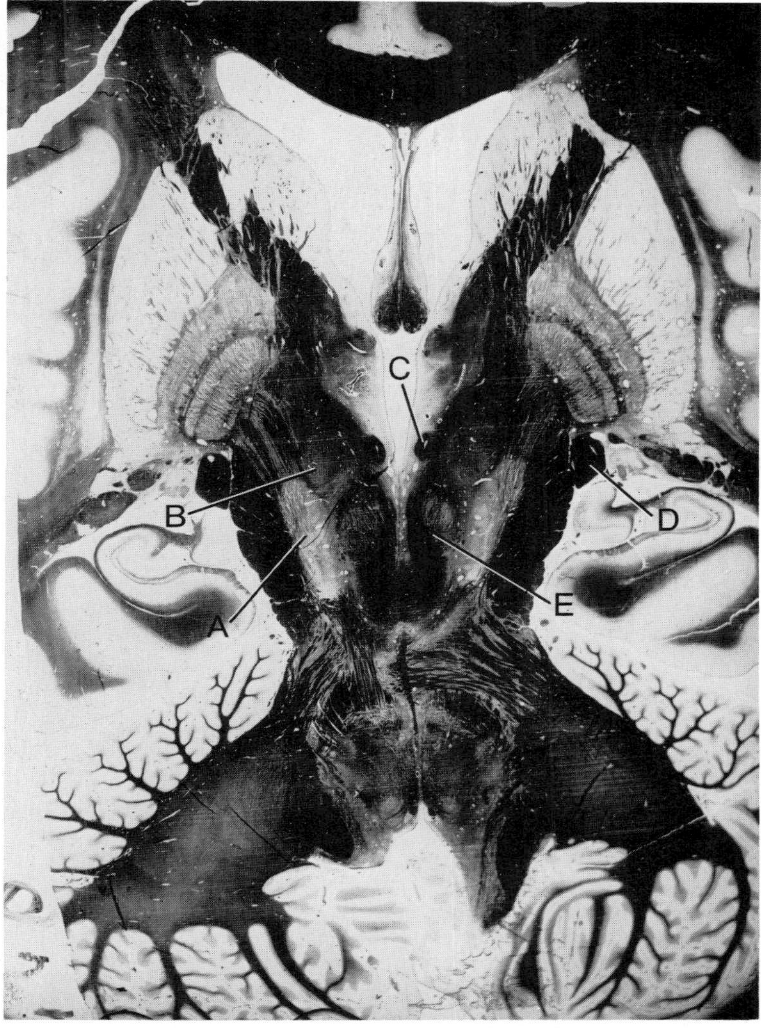

Figure 9.5. Horizontal section in the axis of the brain stem (Weigert's myelin stain). (From H. A. Riley, *Atlas of the Basal Ganglia, Brain Stem and Spinal Cord*, 1943; courtesy of Williams & Wilkins, Baltimore.)

9.44. Red nucleus

9.45. Subthalamic nucleus

9.46. Source of striatal dopamine

9.47. Optic tract

For each numbered item, select the lettered structure in Fig. 9.6 most closely associated with it. Each lettered structure may be selected once, more than once or not at all.

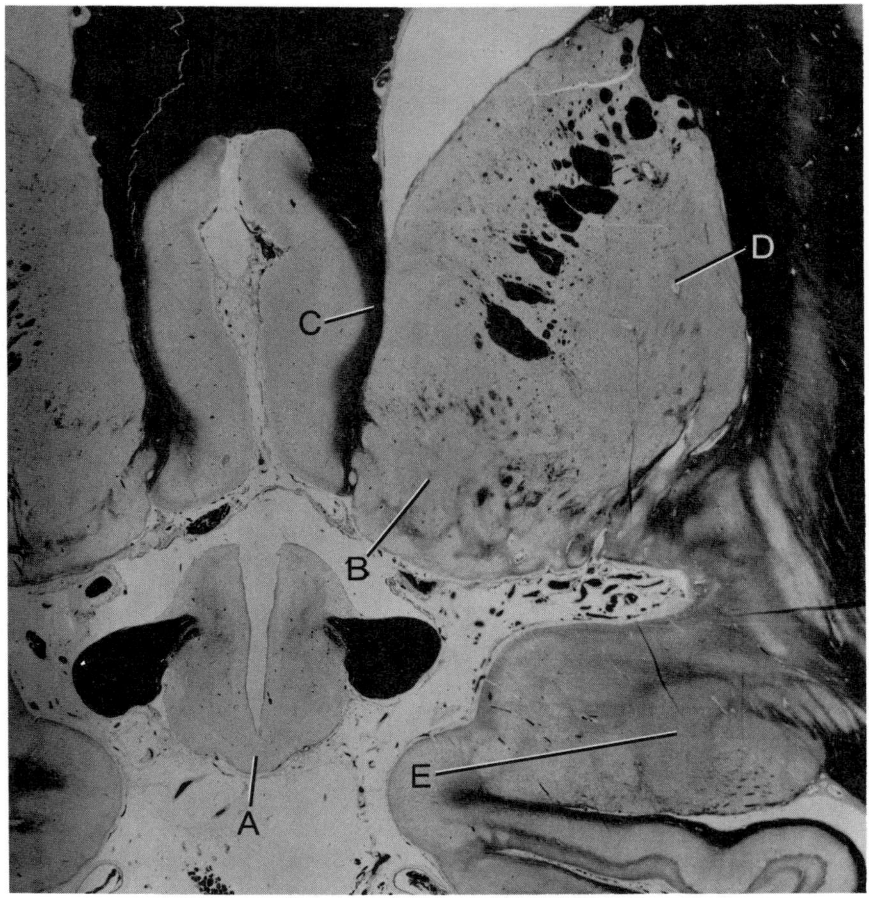

Figure 9.6. Transverse section through forebrain and part of diencephalon (Weigert's myelin stain). (From H. A. Riley, *Atlas of the Basal Ganglia, Brain Stem and Spinal Cord,* 1943; courtesy of Williams & Wilkins, Baltimore.)

9.48. Receptive component of the corpus striatum

9.49. Nucleus accumbens septi

9.50. Portions of this structure project fibers to hypothalamus and neostriatum

9.51. Median eminence

For each numbered item, indicate whether it is associated with

A only (A)
B only (B)
Both A and B (C)
Neither A or B (D)

Questions 9.52–9.55

(A) Medial pallidal segment
(B) Lateral pallidal segment
(C) Both
(D) Neither

9.52. Receive(s) projections from the subthalamic nucleus

9.53. Receive(s) cortical projections

9.54. Project(s) to the subthalamic nucleus

9.55. Transmit(s) γ-aminobutyric acid (GABA) to pars compacta of substantia nigra

Questions 9.56–9.59

(A) Spiny striatal neurons
(B) Aspiny striatal neurons
(C) Both
(D) Neither

9.56. Striatal interneurons

9.57. Receive(s) terminal projections of striatal afferents

9.58. Project(s) fibers to globus pallidus and pars reticulata of substantia nigra

9.59. Project(s) axons to thalamic relay nuclei

Questions 9.60–9.63

(A) Receives cortical projections
(B) Projects to cerebral cortex
(C) Both
(D) Neither

9.60. Subthalamic nucleus

9.61. Substantia nigra

9.62. Neostriatum

9.63. Globus pallidus

Questions 9.64–9.67

(A) Medial pallidal segment
(B) Substantia nigra, pars reticulata
(C) Both
(D) Neither

9.64. Project(s) fibers to thalamus and midbrain tegmentum

9.65. Receive(s) fibers from cerebral cortex

9.66. Derived from diencephalic anlage

9.67. Major input(s) derived from striatum

For each of the incomplete statements below, *one* or *more* of the completions given is correct. Choose answer:

(A) Only **1, 2,** and **3** are correct
(B) Only **1** and **3** are correct
(C) Only **2** and **4** are correct
(D) Only **4** is correct
(E) **All** are correct

9.68. The substantia nigra receives:
(1) a serotonergic (5-HT) projection from the dorsal nucleus of raphe nucleus
(2) strionigral fibers that convey substance P (undecapeptide)
(3) strionigral and pallidonigral projections that have GABA as their neurotransmitter
(4) dopaminergic fibers from the neostriatum

9.69. Abnormal involuntary movement (dyskinesia) associated with pathology of the corpus striatum and related nuclei:
(1) is considered of the physiological expression of "release phenomena"
(2) partially depends upon pallidothalamic projections
(3) is dependent upon the integrity of the motor cortex and the corticospinal system
(4) occurs contralateral to lesions

9.70. The neostriatum:
(1) receives fibers from all cortical areas
(2) has reciprocal connections with the substantia nigra
(3) constitutes the receptive part of the corpus striatum
(4) receives input from intralaminar thalamic nuclei

9.71. Structures projecting fibers to the globus pallidus include:
(1) motor cortex
(2) putamen
(3) red nucleus
(4) subthalamic nucleus

9.72. Reciprocal connections exist between:
(1) the substantia nigra and the neostriatum
(2) the subthalamic nucleus and the globus pallidus
(3) the granular frontal cortex and the dorsomedial nucleus
(4) VLo and the primary motor cortex

9.73. Dopamine:
(1) is transported to all parts of the neostriatum
(2) is synthesized in the olfactory bulb
(3) inhibits prolactin release
(4) is synthesized in the pars compacta of the substantia nigra

9.74. The corpus striatum and the limbic system are considered to be interrelated functionally because:
(1) parts of the amygdaloid nucleus complex project to the neostriatum
(2) they have common neurotransmitters
(3) the medial pallidal segment projects to the lateral habenular nucleus
(4) they have similar behavioral correlates

9.75. The pars reticulata of the substantia nigra projects fibers to:
(1) ventral anterior thalamic nucleus, parvicellular part (VApc)
(2) ventral anterior thalamic nucleus, magnocellular part (VAmc)
(3) ventral lateral thalamic nucleus, pars oralis (VLo)
(4) dorsomedial thalamic nucleus, pars paralaminaris (DMpl)

9.76. Inputs to the neostriatum arise from:
(1) virtually all neocortical areas
(2) the basal lateral amygdala
(3) the phylogenetically oldest thalamic nuclei
(4) the dorsal nucleus of the raphe

9.77. Horseradish peroxidase (HRP) injected into the neostriatum of an animal would retrogradely label neurons in the:
(1) V layer of the cerebral cortex
(2) centromedian nucleus of the thalamus
(3) pars compacta of the substantia nigra
(4) medial pallidal segment

9.78. Injection of kainic acid into the neostriatum of an animal would:

(1) significantly reduce striatal glutamic acid decarboxylase (GAD)
(2) diminish striatal choline acetyltransferase
(3) produce no changes in striatal dopamine
(4) produce cell changes in the cells of the substantia nigra

9.79. The medial pallidal segment projects fibers to the:

(1) subthalamic nucleus
(2) substantia nigra
(3) raphe nuclei
(4) pedunculopontine nucleus

9.80. Dyskinesia (abnormal involuntary movement) due to lesions involving the corpus striatum and related nuclei:

(1) occurs contralateral to the lesions
(2) disappears during sleep
(3) is exaggerated by excitement and self-consciousness
(4) invariably is associated with some degree of paresis

Answers and Explanations*

9.1. **E** The globus pallidus is a diencephalic derivative. See p. 290

9.2. **D** Nigrostriatal and strionigral fibers are reciprocal but arise from, and terminate in, different parts of the substantia nigra

9.3. **E** Collaterals of pallidothalamic fibers end in the centromedian nucleus

9.4. **B** See p. 319

9.5. **C** See p. 318

9.6. **D** See p. 318

9.7. **C** See pp. 298–300

9.8. **D** Glutamate is the neurotransmitter of corticostriate projections

9.9. **C** Neither tyrosine hydroxylase (T-OH) or dopamine are reduced in the striatum in the brains of patients with Huntington's disease

9.10. **D** Thalamic projections from the substantia nigra, the deep cerebellar nuclei, and the globus pallidus terminate in distinctive nuclei. The ventral lateral nucleus of the thalamus (VLo) receives pallidal efferents and projects to the premotor (and supplementary) area

9.11. **D** See p. 301

9.12. **C** See p. 300

9.13. **E** The best evidence suggests that dopamine has a weak excitatory effect upon striatal neurons. See p. 301

9.14. **B** See pp. 301–303

9.15. **B** See pp. 310 and 315

9.16. **D** Collaterals of some cells in the pars reticulata project to both thalamus (VAmc, VLm, and DMpl) and superior colliculus. See p. 311

9.17. **C** See p. 308

9.18. **E** See pp. 298–301

9.19. **E** See p. 298 and Fig. 11-11

9.20. **A** See p. 307 and Figs. 11-14, 11-15, 11-16, and 11-17

9.21. **B** The prefrontal cortex projects ipsilaterally to multiple parts of the caudate nucleus. See p. 299

9.22. **C** Fornix. See p. 337

9.23. **E** See p. 320

9.24. **A** See pp. 167 and 301

9.25. **D** Substance P is found in the striatum, pallidum substantia nigra brain stem nuclei, spinal cord, and spinal ganglia

9.26. **C** See p. 295 and Fig. 11-10

9.27. **E** Zona incerta separates these fibers

9.28. **C** Subthalamic nucleus neurons, see p. 306

9.29. **B**

9.30. **D** Substantia nigra

9.31. **C** Tremor at rest is one feature that characterizes paralysis agitans

9.32. **A** See p. 320

9.33. **D** See p. 218

9.34. **B** A lesion in the subthalamic nucleus or an injection of a γ-aminobutyric acid antagonist into the subthalamic nucleus produces contralateral hemiballism, due to removal of inhibitory influences acting on the medial pallidal segment. See p. 321

9.35. **D** Structure is subthalamic nucleus

9.36. **A** Kainic acid, an analogue of glutamic acid, is a neurotoxin which destroys cells, but not fibers of passage. Such an injection in the striatum destroys spiny neurons

9.37. **A** HRP injected into the striatum would label cells of afferents projecting to it. Such an injection would also label cells of the dorsal nucleus of the raphe

* All page numbers and illustration citations refer to Carpenter: CORE TEXT OF NEUROANATOMY, 3rd edition; © 1985, Williams & Wilkins.

9.38. **B** Structure is lateral pallidal segment which receives fibers and terminals of GABAergic and enkephalin containing striatal projections

9.39. **C** Medial pallidal segment receives spiny striatal projections containing these neurotransmitters. See Fig. 11-10

9.40. **B** Double fluorescent retrograde labeling technics indicate most cells of the subthalamic nucleus project to both the globus pallidus and the pars reticulata of the substantia nigra

9.41. **D** Cells in centromedian nucleus project predominantly to the putamen, but have collaterals which end in the cerebral cortex

9.42. **A** Structure is substantia nigra. Some cells in pars reticulata project to VAmc, VLm and DMpl and the middle gray layers of the superior colliculus

9.43. **E** Structure is red nucleus

9.44. **E**

9.45. **B**

9.46. **A** Structure is the substantia nigra

9.47. **D**

9.48. **D** Neostriatum

9.49. **B** One of the septal nuclei closely related to neostriatum

9.50. **E** Amygdala. See p. 300

9.51. **A** See p. 279 and Fig. 10-15

9.52. **C** Both pallidal segments receive afferents from the subthalamic nucleus

9.53. **D** Neither pallidal segment receives afferent from the cerebral cortex

9.54. **B** Only the lateral pallidal segment projects to the subthalamic nucleus

9.55. **B** The lateral pallidal segment projects GABAergic fibers to the pars compacta of the substantia nigra. See p. 311

9.56. **B** See Fig. 11-10

9.57. **A** See p. 300

9.58. **A** See pp. 301–303

9.59. **D**

9.60. **A** See Fig. 11-23

9.61. **D**

9.62. **C** Projections from cerebral cortex to neostriatum are massive while those from neostriatum to cortex are very small

9.63. **D** Unlike the neostriatum the paleostriatum neither receives or projects fibers to the cerebral cortex

9.64. **C** See Fig. 11-24

9.65. **D**

9.66. **A**

9.67. **C** See Figs. 11-10 and 11-22

9.68. **A**

9.69. **E** See p. 322

9.70. **E**

9.71. **C**

9.72. **A**

9.73. **E** See Fig. 11-10 and pp. 282 and 325

9.74. **B** See pp. 225 and 300

9.75. **C** See Fig. 7-18

9.76. **E**

9.77. **A** See pp. 298–300

9.78. **A** See p. 320

9.79. **D** See p. 310

9.80. **A** See pp. 318–322

10

Olfactory Pathways, Hippocampal Formation, and Amygdala

Questions

Select the one best answer

10.1. Olfactory impulses are relayed directly to the cerebral cortex by the:
- (A) anterior olfactory nucleus
- (B) anterior nuclear group of the thalamus
- (C) subiculum
- (D) dentate gyrus
- (E) lateral olfactory stria

10.2. Experimental studies, in which animals can deliver electrical stimuli to regions of their own brain by bar pressing, suggest that such stimuli:
- (A) damage the brains of animals
- (B) lead to hypersexuality
- (C) represent a primary reinforcement for drives related to food and sex
- (D) are commonly unpleasant and lead to avoidance reactions
- (E) produce neurotic animals

10.3. The following are true concerning the hippocampus, *except*:
- (A) it receives most of its afferents from the entorhinal cortex
- (B) it receives afferents from the septal region
- (C) it projects to the anterior nuclei of the thalamus
- (D) it is involved in olfaction
- (E) it is implicated in memory imprinting

10.4. The amygdaloid nuclear complex:
- (A) has direct connections from the tail of the caudate nucleus
- (B) receives primary and secondary olfactory fibers, but is not essential for olfactory discrimination
- (C) gives rise to major fibers in the anterior commissure
- (D) is essential for olfactory discrimination
- (E) is concerned with recent memory

10.5. The neural structure considered to be most concerned with recent memory is the:
- (A) frontal lobe
- (B) dominant parietal lobe
- (C) hippocampal formation
- (D) mammillary bodies
- (E) amygdaloid complex

10.6. The "limbic" lobe includes all of the following, *except* the:
- (A) cingulate gyrus
- (B) paracentral lobule
- (C) parahippocampal gyrus
- (D) subcallosal gyrus
- (E) hippocampus

10.7. The corticomedial amygdala:
(A) does not receive direct olfactory fibers
(B) projects to the lateral hypothalamus
(C) projects to the thalamus via the ventral amygdalofugal pathway
(D) projects to the ventromedial hypothalamus via the stria terminalis
(E) projects to the hippocampus

10.8. Olfactory receptors:
(A) are unipolar neurons
(B) lie in the olfactory bulb
(C) have a life span of 30–40 days
(D) give rise to myelinated fibers
(E) are of several morphological types

10.9. Primary olfactory fibers synapse upon:
(A) mitral cells
(B) granule cells
(C) descending dendrites of mitral cells
(D) cells of the anterior olfactory nucleus
(E) tufted cells

10.10. Mitral cells in the olfactory bulb send axons or collaterals, to the following, *except*:
(A) olfactory tubercle (anterior perforated substance)
(B) prepyriform cortex
(C) corticomedial amygdala
(D) hippocampal formation
(E) anterior olfactory nucleus

10.11. The prepyriform cortex projects fibers to all of the following, *except*:
(A) entorhinal cortex
(B) dorsomedial thalamus
(C) basolateral amygdala
(D) hippocampal formation
(E) nucleus of the diagonal band

10.12. The amygdaloid nucleus complex receives afferents from all of the following, *except*:
(A) parabrachial nuclei
(B) raphe nuclei
(C) hypothalamus
(D) entorhinal cortex
(E) locus ceruleus

For each numbered item, select the one heading most closely associated with it. Each lettered heading may be selected once, more than once, or not at all.

Questions 10.13–10.16

(A) Psalterium
(B) Papez's theory of emotion
(C) Korsakoff's syndrome
(D) Klüver-Bucy syndrome
(E) Limbic lobe

10.13. Associated with alcoholism and thiamine deficiency

10.14. Associated with "psychic blindness," bizzare oral and sexual behavior, docility, and change in dietary habits

10.15. Hippocampal (fornical) commissure

10.16. Consists of archicortex, paleocortex, and juxtallocortex

Questions 10.17–10.20

(A) Opiate receptors
(B) Dopamine
(C) Raphe nuclei
(D) Enkephalin, substance P, and somatostatin
(E) Choline acetyltransferase

10.17. Terminals containing this neurotransmitter are densest in the central nucleus of the amygdala

10.18. Contained mainly in central and medial amygdaloid nuclei

10.19. Distributed throughout amygdala, except for lateral nucleus

10.20. Fibers containing this transmitter originate from the ventral tegmental area

For each numbered item, select the lettered structure most closely associated with it in Fig. 10.1. Each lettered structure may be selected once, more than once, or not at all.

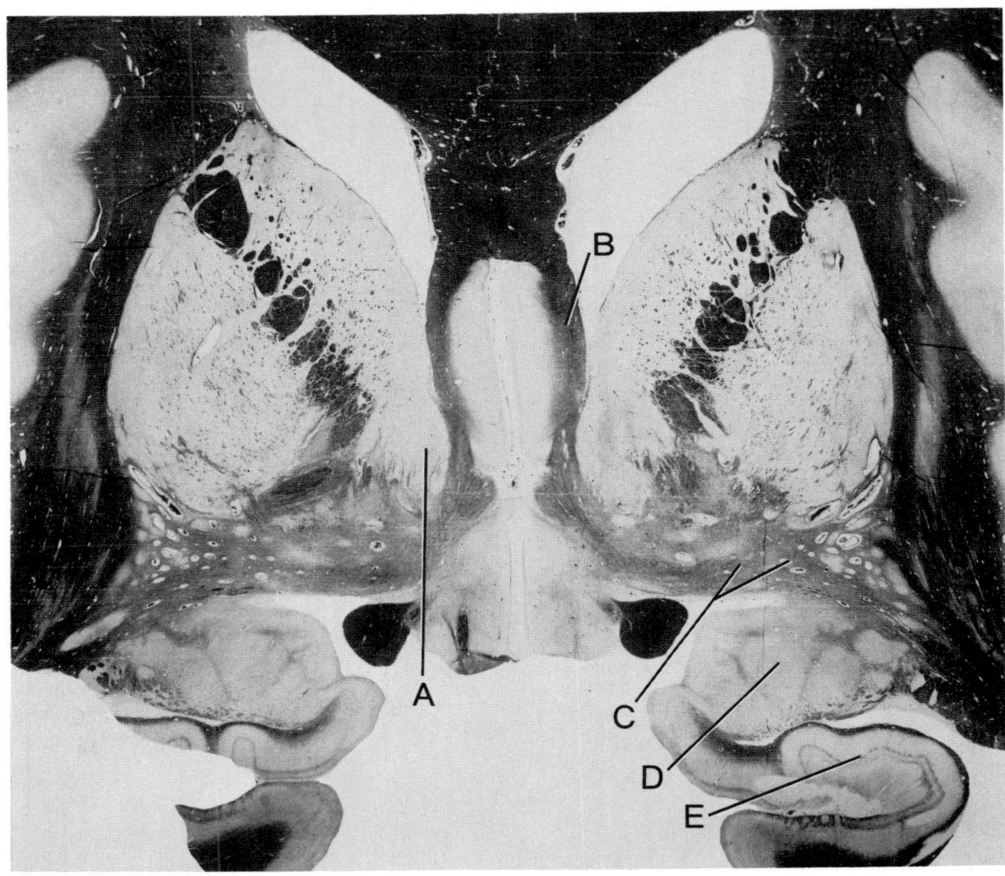

Figure 10.1. Transverse section of forebrain perpendicular to the longitudinal axis of the brain stem. (From H. A. Riley, *Atlas of the Basal Ganglia, Brain Stem and Spinal Cord*, 1943; courtesy of Williams & Wilkins.)

10.21. Concerned with behavioral, visceral, and endocrine functions

10.22. Part of a massive commissural system

10.23. Large cells distribute cholinergic fibers widely in the cerebral cortex

10.24. The septal nucleus most closely related to the corpus striatum

For each numbered item, select the one heading most closely associated with it. Each lettered heading may be selected once, more than once, or not at all.

Questions 10.25–10.28

(A) Subiculum
(B) Choroid fissure
(C) Parahippocampal gyrus
(D) Fasciolar gyrus
(E) Dentate gyrus

10.25. Includes the entorhinal cortex

10.26. Located on the ventral lip of the hippocampal fissure

10.27. Extends onto the superior surface of the corpus callosum as the indusium griseum

10.28. Exposed by separating the lips of the hippocampal fissure

For each numbered item, select the letter designating the part in Fig. 10.2. which matches it correctly. A lettered part may be selected once, more than once, or not at all.

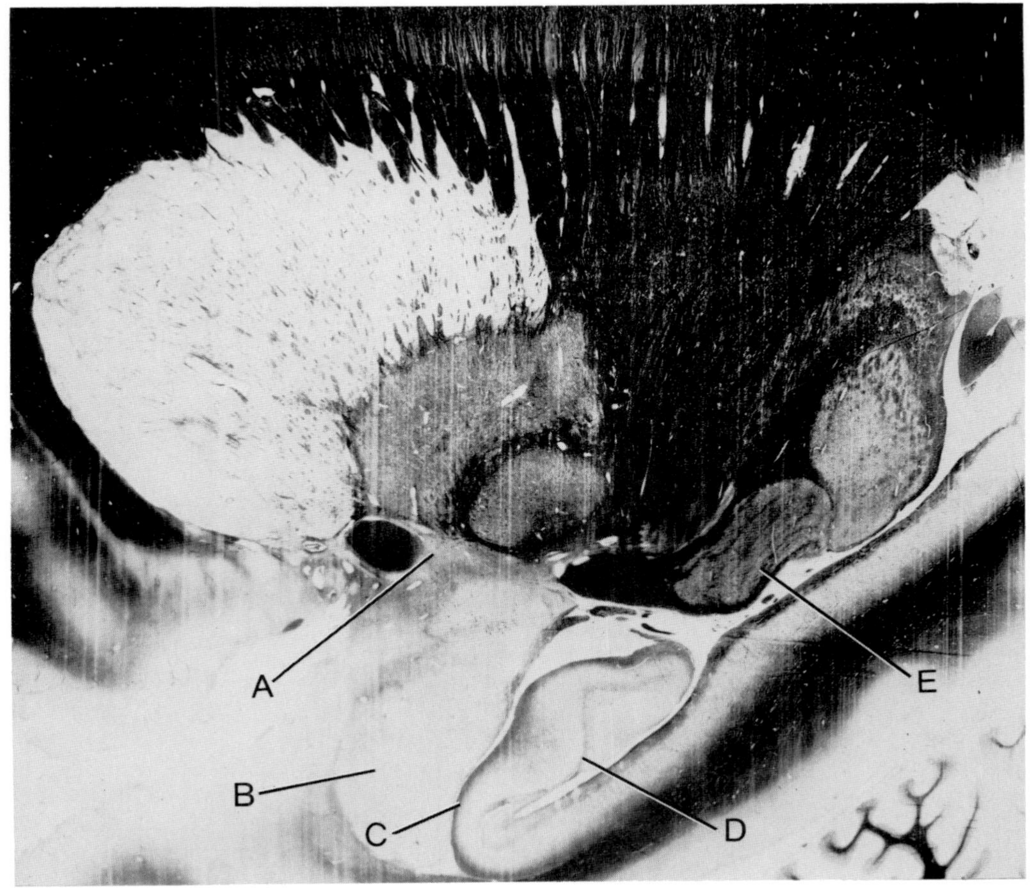

Figure 10.2. Sagittal section through the basal ganglia and inferior horn of the lateral ventricle. (From H. A. Riley, *Atlas of the Basal Ganglia, Brain Stem and Spinal Cord*, 1943; courtesy of Williams & Wilkins.)

10.29. Alveus

10.30. Dentate gyrus

10.31. Substantia innominata

10.32. Amygdaloid nuclear complex

For each numbered item, indicate whether it is associated with

A only (A)
B only (B)
Both A and B (C)
Neither A or B (D)

Questions 10.33–10.36

(A) Primary olfactory cortex
(B) Secondary olfactory cortex
(C) Both
(D) Neither

10.33. Receives fibers from prepyriform cortex

10.34. Received afferents from the lateral olfactory stria

10.35. Forms the pyriform lobe

10.36. Projects to the hippocampal formation

Questions 10.37–10.40

(A) Primary olfactory pathway
(B) Somesthetic pathway
(C) Both
(D) Neither

10.37. Specific thalamocortical relay

10.38. Somatotopical organized

10.39. Polysynaptic influence upon hippocampal neurons

10.40. Direct projections to hippocampal neurons

Questions 10.41–10.44

(A) Dentate gyrus
(B) Hippocampal formation
(C) Both
(D) Neither

10.41. Archipallium

10.42. Structurally consists of three major cellular layers

10.43. Contains large pyramidal projection neurons

10.44. Contains a prominent granule cell layer

Questions 10.45–10.48

(A) Precommissural fornix
(B) Postcommissural fornix
(C) Both
(D) Neither

10.45. Fibers project to medial mammillary nucleus, and to anterior and rostral intralaminar thalamic nuclei

10.46. Fibers originate from the subiculum

10.47. Distributes fibers to septal nuclei and preoptic area

10.48. Fibers originate from dentate gyrus

Questions 10.49–10.52

(A) Hypothalamus
(B) Amygdala
(C) Both
(D) Neither

10.49. Bilateral lesions are associated with docile behavior

10.50. Associated with mechanisms that control food intake

10.51. Stimulation associated with release of ACTH and gonadotrophic hormone

10.52. Electrical stimulation produces an "arrest" reaction and aroused attention

Questions 10.53–10.56

(A) Septal nuclei
(B) Amygdala
(C) Both
(D) Neither

10.53. Region of interaction of olfactory and extraolfactory inputs

10.54. Output system involves medial forebrain bundle

10.55. Output passes via stria medullaris to habenular nuclei

10.56. Projects to magnocellular part of dorsomedial nucleus

For each of the incomplete statements below, *one* or *more* of the completions given is correct. Choose answer:

(A) Only **1, 2,** and **3** are correct
(B) Only **1** and **3** are correct
(C) Only **2** and **4** are correct
(D) Only **4** is correct
(E) **All** are correct

10.57. The substantia innominata (basal nuclei):
(1) contains cholinergic neurons with widespread cortical projections
(2) has a typical cortical organization
(3) selectively dgenerates in Alzheimer's disease and its variants
(4) is involved in Korsakoff's syndrome

10.58. The stria terminalis:
(1) originates in the corticomedial amygdala
(2) courses in the sulcus at the junction of the thalamus and caudate nucleus
(3) conveys fibers to the ventromedial hypothalamic nucleus
(4) is concerned with recent memory

10.59. The primary olfactory cortex:
(1) includes the uncus and part of the parahippocampal gyrus
(2) is not evident on the surface of the brain
(3) receives the lateral olfactory stria
(4) includes temporal lobe cortex lateral to the collateral and rhinal sulci

10.60. Nuclei playing a significant role in the limbic system include:
(1) amygdaloid nucleus
(2) interpeduncular nucleus
(3) habenular nucleus
(4) centromedian nucleus

10.61. The fornix:
(1) contains efferents from the hippocampal formation and subiculum
(2) projects to the septal region
(3) projects to the mammillary bodies
(4) projects to the anterior and rostral intralaminar thalamic nuclei

10.62. Olfactory receptors:
(1) are bipolar neurons
(2) lie in patch of the nasal epithelium
(3) have central unmyelinated processes, the olfactoria fila
(4) lie in the olfactory bulb

10.63. In the mammillary body:
(1) the lateral nucleus has reciprocal connections with the dorsal and ventral tegmental nuclei
(2) the medial nucleus receives direct inputs from the subiculum
(3) the medial mammillary nucleus projects to the anterior nuclear group of the thalamus
(4) Precommissural fibers terminate in the medial mammillary nucleus

10.64. Olfactory sense can be tested in each nostril by having the patient sniff:
(1) substances which stimulate gustatory receptors
(2) liquids with characteristic odors
(3) irritating volatile oils
(4) camphoraceous substances

10.65. Fibers of the olfactory tract:
(1) represent axons of mitral and tufted cells
(2) axons of granule cells
(3) terminate in pyriform cortex and the corticomedial amygdala
(4) end in the entorhinal cortex

10.66. The anterior commissure:
(1) contains interconnections between the anterior olfactory nuclei
(2) contains interconnections between the middle and inferior temporal gyri
(3) traverses ventral parts of the lateral pallidal segment
(4) laterally blends with the external capsule

10.67. Reciprocal synapses occur:
(1) in olfactory glomeruli
(2) in the anterior olfactory nucleus
(3) in the corticomedial amygdala
(4) between granule and mitral cell dendrites

10.68. Clinically Alzheimer's disease and its variants are characterized by:
(1) loss of recent memory
(2) confusion and disorientation
(3) slurred speech
(4) confabulation

10.69. Electrical stimulation of the amygdala produces:
(1) autonomic responses
(2) endocrine responses
(3) somatic responses (chewing, licking, and swallowing)
(4) hypersexual behavior

Answers and Explanations*

10.1. E See p. 325

10.2. C see p. 347

10.3. D See p. 338

10.4. B See p. 342

10.5. C See p. 338

10.6. B Paracentral lobule is concerned with somatic motor and sensory functions

10.7. D See pp. 340–341

10.8. C See p. 324

10.9. C See p. 324

10.10. D See p. 325

10.11. D Hippocampal formation receives major input from enorhinal cortex

10.12. D See p. 340

10.13. C See p. 338

10.14. D See p. 344

10.15. A See p. 337

10.16. E See p. 345

10.17. B See p. 340

10.18. D See p. 340

10.19. A See p. 340

10.20. B See p. 340

10.21. D Represents the amygdaloid nuclear complex

10.22. B Represents rostrum of the corpus callosum

10.23. C Represents the substantia innominata

10.24. A Represents the nucleus accumbens septi

10.25. C The rostrolateral part of the parahippocampal gyrus represents the entorhinal cortex (Bodmann's area 28). See Fig. 12-12

10.26. A See Fig. 12-10

10.27. D See Fig. 12-8 and p. 333

10.28. E

10.29. C The ventricular surface of the hippocampus is covered by myelinated axons which form the alveus

10.30. D See p. 333

10.31. A See p. 344

10.32. B Representing the corticomedial amygdala

10.33. B See pp. 326–327

10.34. A See p. 325

10.35. C See p. 326

10.36. B See p. 337

10.37. B See p. 261

10.38. B See pp. 242 and 261

10.39. A See p. 337

10.40. D See p. 337

10.41. C See p. 323

10.42. C See pp. 334-335

10.43. B See pp. 334 and 337

10.44. A See pp. 335–337

10.45. B See p. 337

10.46. B See p. 337

10.47 A See p. 338

10.48. D See pp. 335-337

10.49. B See p. 343

10.50. C See pp. 287 and 344

10.51. C See pp. 286 and 343

10.52. B See p. 342

10.53. C See Fig. 12-15

10.54. C See p. 270

10.55. A See p. 329

10.56. B See p. 230

10.57. B See pp. 344-345

10.58. A See pp. 340-341

10.59. B See pp. 325-326

10.60. A See p. 346

10.61. E See pp. 337-338

* All page numbers and illustration citations refer to Carpenter: CORE TEXT OF NEUROANATOMY, 3rd edition; © 1985, Williams & Wilkins.

10.62. A See pp. 323-324
10.63. A See pp. 270-271, 272, 276, and 338
10.64. C See p. 330
10.65. B See p. 325 and Fig. 12-3
10.66. E See pp. 331-332
10.67. D See p. 324; Fig. 12-3
10.68. A See p. 345
10.69. A See p. 343

11

Cerebral Cortex

Questions

Select the one best answer

11.1. The most massive projection from the cerebral cortex terminates in the:
- (A) neostriatum
- (B) thalamic nuclei
- (C) spinal cord
- (D) pontine nuclei
- (E) superior colliculus

11.2. Binocular fusion in the visual system first occurs in:
- (A) laminae 1, 4, and 6 of the lateral geniculate body
- (B) laminae 2, 3, and 5 of the lateral geniculate body
- (C) layer 4 of the primary visual cortex
- (D) layers above and below layer 4 in the primary visual cortex
- (E) the bilaminar segment

11.3. A large lesion in the region of the transverse gyri of Heschl would:
- (A) impair hearing only contralaterally
- (B) impair hearing bilaterally, with the greatest loss contralaterally
- (C) produce auditory hallucinations
- (D) impair sound localization
- (E) impair perception of certain auditory frequencies

11.4. Transient "grasp" reflexes often are seen following ablations, or lesions of, the:
- (A) primary motor area (M I)
- (B) primary somesthetic cortex (S I)
- (C) supplementary motor area
- (D) paleocerebellum
- (E) prefrontal cortex

11.5. A lesion in the inferior frontal gyrus involving the pars triangularis and opercularis of the dominant hemisphere would produce:
- (A) a hemiplegia contralaterally
- (B) loss of recent memory
- (C) impairment of motor aspects of speech
- (D) dysarthria
- (E) impaired audition

11.6. Ablation of the postcentral gyrus unilateral would produce:
- (A) contralateral loss of pain and thermal sense
- (B) abnormal cutaneous sensations contralaterally
- (C) enduring impairment of contralateral kinesthetic and discriminatory tactile sense
- (D) depressed contralateral myotatic reflexes
- (E) enduring loss of all deep and superficial sensation contralaterally

11.7. Cells of the lateral geniculate body project to which layer of the striate cortex (area 17):
- (A) layer VI
- (B) layer III
- (C) layer V
- (D) layer IV
- (E) layer II

For each numbered item select the lettered area (*shaded*) in Fig. 11.1 most closely associated with it. Each lettered area may be selected once, more than once, or not at all.

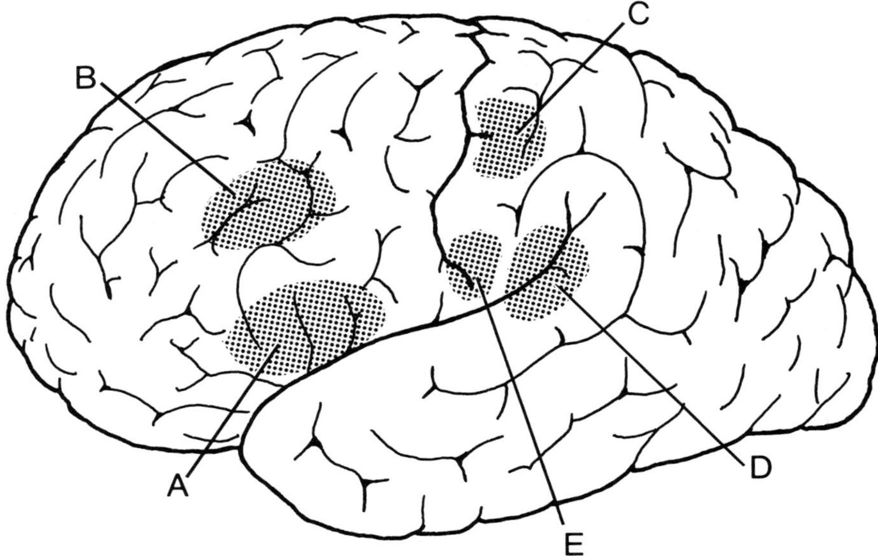

Figure 11.1. Diagram of the lateral convexity of the brain with *shaded areas* repesenting cortical lesions.

11.8. Lesion would impair gustatory sense

11.9. Lesion would produce unequal, but bilateral sensory loss

11.10. Center for voluntary conjugate eye movements, independent of visual input

11.11. In dominant hemisphere lesion would impair speech

For each numbered item, select the one heading most closely associated with it. Each lettered heading may be selected once, more than once, or not at all.

Questions 11.12–11.15

(A) Cortical layer I
(B) Cortical layers II and III
(C) Cortical layer IV
(D) Cortical layer V
(E) Cortical layer VI

11.12. Origin of commissural projections

11.13. Cortical layer receiving most specific sensory inputs

11.14. Corticothalamic projections

11.15. Corticostriate fibers

Questions 11.16–11.19

(A) Allocortex
(B) Homotypical cortex
(C) Koniocortex
(D) Agranular cortex
(E) Juxtallocortex

11.16. Granular cortex characteristic of primary sensory areas

11.17. Premotor and motor cortex

11.18. Typical six layered cortex

11.19. Transitional cortex of cingulate gyrus

Questions 11.20–11.23

(A) Ventral posterior thalamic nucleus
(B) Ventral posteromedial nucleus, pars parvicellularis (VPMpc)
(C) Lateral geniculate nucleus
(D) Inferior pulvinar
(E) Dorsal and medial subdivisions of medial geniculate body

11.20. Projects fibers to parietal operculum, area 43

11.21. Projects to primary (S I) and secondary (SS II) somesthetic cortex

11.22. Projects mainly upon area 17

11.23. Projects upon areas 18 and 19

Questions 11.24–11.27

(A) Cells in laminae 1 and 2 of lateral geniculate body
(B) Cells in laminae 3, 4, 5, and 6 of lateral geniculate body
(C) All cell laminae of lateral geniculate body
(D) "Complex" cells of striate cortex
(E) Simple cells of striate cortex

11.24. Have binocular receptive field properties

11.25. Project fibers to lamina IV of striate cortex

11.26. Receive projections from all laminae of the striate cortex

11.27. Project to the suprachiasmatic nucleus, the superior colliculus, and the pretectum

Questions 11.28–11.31

(A) Area 3
(B) Area 2
(C) Area 1
(D) Area 3a
(E) Area 5

11.28. Located in the depth of the central sulcus and considered to receive input from stretch receptors

11.29. Postulated to represent the "command center" for limb and hand movements

11.30. Over 90% of cell columns are related to receptors in deep tissue

11.31. Majority of cell columns respond to cutaneous stimuli

Questions 11.32–11.35

(A) Primary motor area (M I)
(B) Premotor area
(C) Supplementary motor area (M II)
(D) Paracentral lobule
(E) Primary somesthetic area (S I)

11.32. Stimulation produces bilateral responses of a tonic and postural nature

11.33. Contains motor and sensory representation of the contralateral lower extremity

11.34. Provides inputs to the primary motor area (M I) and the supplementary motor area (M II)

11.35. Has no clear-cut cytoarchitectonic borders

Questions 11.36–11.39

(A) Retinal ganglion cells
(B) "Simple cells" in striate cortex
(C) "Complex cells" in striate cortex
(D) Superficial layers of superior colliculus
(E) Cells in the parabigeminal nucleus

11.36. Receive monocular inputs from the lateral geniculate body

11.37. Respond to small stationary spots of light

11.38. Respond to both moving and stationary spots of light

11.39. Respond to moving stimuli in visual field with preferred directional selectivity

For each numbered item, indicate whether it is associated with

A only (A)
B only (B)
Both A and B (C)
Neither A or B (D)

Questions 11.40–11.43

(A) Dominant hemisphere
(B) Nondominant hemisphere
(C) Both
(D) Neither

11.40. Related to handedness and speech center

11.41. Concerned with spatial concepts, recognition of faces, music, and pictographic language

11.42. Asterognosis

11.43 Rapid eye movements (REM)

Questions 11.44–11.47

(A) Ocular dominance columns
(B) Orientation columns
(C) Both
(D) Neither

11.44. Only partially formed at birth

11.45. Associated with representation of the blind spot

11.46. Innately determined and not modified by visual deprivation

11.47. Extends throughout all layers of the striate cortex

Questions 11.48–11.51.

(A) "Simple cells" in striate cortex
(B) "Complex cells" in striate cortex
(C) Both
(D) Neither

11.48. Respond to small flickering spots of light

11.49. Receive input from sets of lateral geniculate neurons whose "on" or "off" centers form a line corresponding to the orientation axis

11.50. Exhibit both ocular dominance and binocular qualities

11.51. Exhibit varying receptive field orientation and alternating monocular responses

Questions 11.52–11.55

(A) Primary motor cortex (M I)
(B) Premotor cortex
(C) Both
(D) Neither

11.52. Contains giant pyramidal cells

11.53. Classified as agranular frontal cortex

11.54. Layer V contributes fibers to the corticospinal tract

11.55. Projects bilaterally and somatotopically upon portions of the putamen

Questions 11.56–11.59

(A) Area 17
(B) Area 18
(C) Both
(D) Neither

11.56. Representation of the contralateral visual hemifield, or major central parts of it

11.57. Stereoscopic depth perception

11.58. Cell columns respond to slits of light, dark bars and edges with specific orientations

11.59. Vertical meridian of visual field is represented bilaterally because of commissural connections

Questions 11.60–11.63

(A) Primary auditory cortex (A I)
(B) Secondary auditory cortex (A II)
(C) Both
(D) Neither

11.60. Receives input from the laminated subdivision of the medial geniculate body

11.61. Receive thalamic projections via the sublenticular portion of the internal capsule

11.62. Projects commissural fibers to contralateral auditory areas

11.63. Constitutes the auditory cortical "belt"

For each numbered item in Fig. 11.2, indicate whether it is associated with

A only (A)
B only (B)
Both A and B (C)
Neither A nor B (D)

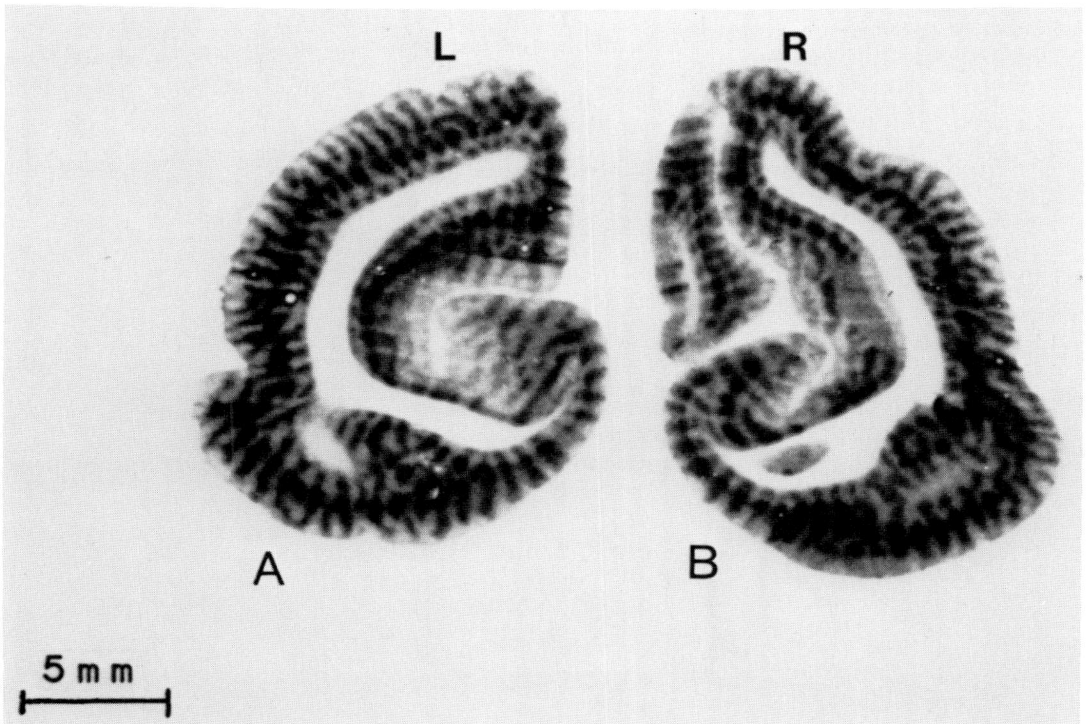

Figure 11.2. 2[^{14}C]Deoxyglucose autoradiographic mapping of left (*L*) and right (*R*) striate cortex of a monkey in which one eye has been enucleated. (Courtesy of Dr. Louis Sokoloff, National Institutes of Health.)

11.64. Ocular dominance columns

11.65. Representation of the monocular visual field

11.66. Representation of the blind spot

11.67. Cortical region which "covers" the blind spot of the enucleated eye

For each numbered item, indicate whether it is associated with

A only (A)
B only (B)
Both A and B (C)
Neither A or B (D)

Questions 11.68–11.71

(A) Vertical encoding
(B) Horizontal encoding
(C) Both
(D) Neither

11.68. Representation of tonal frequency, sensory modality, or receptive axis of orientation in primary sensory areas

11.69. Representation of position in the visual field

11.70. Binocular fusion in striate cortex

11.71. Cerebral dominance

Instructions for Questions 11.72–11.90

For each of the incomplete statements below, *one* or *more* of the completions given is correct. Choose answer:

(A) Only **1, 2,** and **3** are correct
(B) Only **1** and **3** are correct
(C) Only **2** and **4** are correct
(D) Only **4** is correct
(E) **All** are correct

11.72. The supplementary motor area of the cerebral cortex is:

(1) located on the medial aspect of the hemisphere
(2) coextensive with Brodmann's area 6
(3) part of a bilateral motor system concerned with postural and tonic movements
(4) not somatotopically organized

11.73. The motor homunculus:

(1) is a distorted, inverted somatotopic representation of the body in the precentral gyrus
(2) has representation of various body parts that correspond in area to those of the sensory homunculus
(3) when electrically stimulated gives rise to movements on the opposite side of the body
(4) if parts are ablated, contralateral paralysis develops in corresponding body regions

11.74. Inputs to the primary motor cortex (area 4) are derived from:

(1) the "cell sparse" zone of the ventral lateral nuclear region of the thalamus
(2) the primary somesthetic area (S I)
(3) the second somatic area (SS II)
(4) the ventral posterolateral nucleus, pars caudalis (VPLc)

11.75. The primary somesthetic cortex (S I):

(1) receives the principal cortical projection from the ventral posterolateral (VPLc) and ventral posteromedial (VPM) thalamic nuclei
(2) consists of three cytologically distinct zones
(3) is composed of vertical cell columns which are modality specific and related to small unchanging receptive fields
(4) projects to the primary motor area (M I), the supplementary motor area and the second somatic area (SS II)

11.76. Direct corticofugal projections from frontal, parietal, occipital and temporal lobes terminate in the:

(1) spinal cord gray matter
(2) neostriatum
(3) substantia nigra
(4) pontine nuclei

11.77. Accommodation for near vision involves:

(1) transmission of visual impulses to the striate cortex
(2) corticofugal fibers projecting to the superior colliculus and pretectum
(3) the visceral nuclei of the oculomotor complex
(4) postganglionic fibers from the ciliary ganglion

11.78. "Simple cells" in the striate cortex:

(1) receive inputs from lateral geniculate neurons
(2) respond to "slits" of light with a specific receptive field axis of orientation
(3) have receptive fields with adjacent "on" and "off" areas
(4) provide inputs to "complex cells"

11.79. Neurons projecting directly to cerebral cortex without thalamic relay include:

(1) mitral cells
(2) nucleus basalis (substantia innominata)
(3) locus ceruleus
(4) raphe nuclei

11.80. The electroencephalographic (EEG) arousal response, characterized by low amplitude, desynchronized cortical activity:

(1) is abolished in the cerveau isolé preparation
(2) can be elicited by stimulation of either the lemniscal systems or the reticular formation in intact animals
(3) is generated in brain stem reticular formation
(4) can be elicited by 6–12 Hz stimulation of the intralaminar nuclei

11.81. In the secondary sensory area (SS II):

(1) the order of body representation is different than in the primary sensory area (S I)
(2) the boundaries are bordered on all sides by the primary sensory area (S I)
(3) input is received from components of the ipsilateral ventral posterior nucleus (VP), and from S I in both hemispheres
(4) ablations produce major sensory disturbances

11.82. The elementary functional unit of the cerebral cortex:

(1) is determined by the laminar segregation of thalamic inputs
(2) consists of a vertical column of cells extending from the white matter to the pial surface
(3) is determined by cytoarchitectonic boundaries
(4) in the sensory cortex consists of cells related to the same receptive field and same sensory modality

11.83. In the cerebral cortex:

(1) horizontal lamination serves to segregate projection systems
(2) vertical columns form the integrated functional units
(3) Golgi type II interrelate the functional units regionally
(4) commissural projections interrelated cell columns of homologous areas in the two hemispheres

11.84. Neurons with specific neurotransmitters projecting to broad areas of the cerebral cortex arise from:

(1) locus ceruleus
(2) rostral raphe nuclei
(3) nucleus basalis (substantia innominata)
(4) reticular nucleus of the thalamus

11.85. The secondary visual area (V II):

(1) is a mirror image representation of visual area I
(2) receives inputs from the inferior pulvinar and larger cells of lateral geniculate body
(3) has a representation of the vertical meridian of the visual field at its junction with area 17
(4) processes visual information concerned with stereoscopic depth perception

11.86. Secondary sensory areas:

(1) lie adjacent to primary sensory areas
(2) are not somatotopically or topographically organized
(3) receive inputs from the primary sensory area, thalamic nuclei, or both
(4) subserve the same function as the adjacent primary sensory area

11.87. Deprivation of vision in one eye during the first 6 weeks of life may result in:

(1) permanently impaired binocular vision
(2) modifications of striate orientation columns
(3) diminished ocular dominance columns related to the occluded eye
(4) enlargement of the blind spot

11.88. Extrageniculate visual pathways involve:

(1) superior colliculus
(2) parabigeminal nucleus
(3) inferior pulvinar
(4) primarily the striate cortex

11.89. The contralateral visual hemifield is retinotopically represented in:

(1) the inferior pulvinar and adjacent lateral pulvinar
(2) superficial layers of the superior colliculus
(3) the striate cortex
(4) parabigeminal nucleus

11.90. The primary motor cortex (M I):

(1) is somatotopically arranged in the form of the motor homunculus
(2) is electrically excitable with the lowest threshold in the face area
(3) when ablated in primates and man, produces initially a flaccid paralysis, hypotonia and loss of myotatic reflexes contralaterally
(4) when ablated selectively produces paralysis and spasticity

Answers and Explanations*

11.1. D See pp. 135, 197, and 386

11.2. D See pp. 369–370

11.3. B See pp. 376–377

11.4. C See p. 382

11.5. C See pp. 23 and 390

11.6. C See p. 361

11.7. D See pp. 367–368

11.8. E Projections of VPMpc are to the cortex of the parietal operculum; see p. 377

11.9. D A lesion in the primary auditory cortex impairs audition bilaterally with the greatest loss contralaterally; see p. 376

11.10 B The frontal eye field lies in the caudal part of the middle frontal gyrus; see p. 384

11.11. A Broca's speech area lies in the caudal part of the inferior frontal gyrus; see p. 23

11.12. B See p. 353

11.13. C See p. 352

11.41. E See pp. 353 and 386

11.15. D Corticostriate fibers arise from small and medium-sized cells in the upper half of lamina V; see p. 300

11.16. C Koniocortex (dust-like) composed of small granular cells characterizes the primary sensory areas; see p. 373

11.17. D See p. 381

11.18. B See p. 355

11.19. E See p. 345

11.20. B See pp. 244 and 377

11.21. A See pp. 244 and 359

11.22. C See pp. 258 and 362

11.23. D See pp. 239 and 373

11.24. D See p. 371

11.25. B See p. 249

11.26. C See p. 251

11.27. A See pp. 247 and 386

11.28. D See p. 360

11.29. E See p. 384

11.30. B See p. 360

11.31. A See p. 360

11.32. C See p. 381

11.33. D See p. 27

11.34. E See p. 384

11.35. C See p. 383

11.36. B See p. 367

11.37. A See pp. 258 and 363, also Fig. 13-10

11.38. E See p. 173

11.39. D See p. 179

11.40. A See p. 387

11.41. B See p. 388

11.42. C See p. 388

11.43. D REM occur independently of cerebral dominance and are dependent upon projections from the medial vestibular nuclei; see p. 389

11.44. A See p. 372

11.45. D See p. 371; Figs. 13-14, 13-15, and 13-16

11.46. B See p. 372

11.47. C See pp. 366–372

11.48. D See p. 366

11.49. A See p. 366

11.50. B See p. 369–372

11.51. A See pp. 366–368

11.52. A See p. 378

11.53. C See p. 381

11.54. C See p. 379

11.55. A See pp. 298–300

11.56. C See pp. 363–372

11.57. B See p. 373

11.58. C See pp. 363 and 373

* All page numbers and illustration citations refer to Carpenter: CORE TEXT OF NEUROANATOMY, 3rd edition; © 1985, Williams & Wilkins.

11.59. C See p. 373
11.60. A See p. 374
11.61. C See pp. 255 and 373
11.62. C See p. 376
11.63. B See pp. 246 and 375
11.64. C See Fig. 13-14
11.65. D See p. 371
11.66. C See Figs. 13-14, 13-15, and 13-16
11.67. A See Figs. 13-14, 13-15, and 13-16
11.68. A See pp. 360, 368, and 375
11.69. D Surface coordinates (i.e., eccentricity from the fovea and distance above or below the horizontal meridian) determine the topographical position in visual field representation; see p. 366
11.70. B See p. 369
11.71. D See p. 387
11.72. B See pp. 381–383
11.73. E See p. 380
11.74. A See p. 383
11.75. E See p. 359
11.76. C See pp. 135, 197, 298, and 385
11.77. E See p. 185
11.78. E See pp. 366–367
11.79. E See pp. 324–325 and 344
11.80. A See p. 189–190
11.81. B See pp. 361–362
11.82. C See p. 354
11.83. E See pp. 353–354
11.84. A See pp. 252 and 344
11.85. E See pp. 239 and 372
11.86. B See pp. 356–359
11.87. B See p. 372
11.88. B See pp. 239 and 372
11.89. E See pp. 173, 179, 239, 258–260, and 363
11.90. B See pp. 379–380

12

Blood Supply of the Central Nervous System

Questions

Select the one best answer

12.1. Sudden occlusion of one anterior spinal artery near its origin may produce:
- (A) a Brown-Séquard syndrome
- (B) a contralateral hemiparesis and an ipsilateral paralysis of the tongue
- (C) contralateral loss of pain and thermal senses and ipsilateral lower motor neuron symptoms
- (D) paraplegia
- (E) ipsilateral lower motor disturbances

12.2. The blood-cerebrospinal fluid barrier is:
- (A) located in the ependyma
- (B) formed by tight junctions between epithelial cells of the choroid plexus
- (C) due to impermeability of choroid stroma
- (D) equal in surface area to the blood-brain barrier
- (E) due to absence of capillary fenestration

12.3. A cerebral vascular lesion resulting in a contralateral hemiparesis, hemianesthesia, and both motor and sensory aphasia most likely involves branches of:
- (A) the posterior cerebral artery
- (B) the anterior cerebral artery
- (C) the lenticulostriate vessels
- (D) the middle cerebral artery
- (E) the anterior choroidal artery

12.4. The hippocampus, amygdala, and retrolenticular portion of the internal capsule are supplied by the:
- (A) lateral striate arteries
- (B) medial striate artery
- (C) anterior choroidal artery
- (D) posterior choroidal artery
- (E) thalamoperforating arteries

12.5. Sparing of macular vision after occlusion of one posterior cerebral artery may be due to collateral circulation provided by branches of the:
- (A) anterior cerebral artery
- (B) posterior communicating artery
- (C) middle cerebral artery
- (D) superior cerebellar artery
- (E) contralateral posterior cerebral artery

For each numbered item, select the one heading most closely associated with it. Each lettered heading may be selected once, more than once, or not at all.

Questions 12.5–12.9

(A) Middle cerebral artery
(B) Internal carotid artery
(C) Posterior communicating artery
(D) Anterior cerebral artery
(E) Posterior cerebral artery

12.6. Callosomarginal artery

12.7. Calcarine artery

12.8. Ganglionic branches to the anterior hypothalamus

12.9. Striate arteries

Questions 12.10–12.13

(A) Paramedian branches of basilar artery
(B) Anterior inferior cerebellar artery
(C) Anterior spinal artery
(D) Posterior cerebral artery
(E) Bulbar branches of vertebral artery

12.10. Supplies the medullary pyramid and medial lemniscus

12.11. Supplies striate cortex

12.12. Supplies lateral aspect of lower medulla

12.13. Supplies the pontine nuclei and corticospinal tract

Questions 12.14–12.17

(A) Anterior spinal artery
(B) Posterior spinal artery
(C) Posterior inferior cerebellar artery
(D) Superior cerebellar artery
(E) Vertebral artery

12.14. Nuclei gracilis and cuneatus

12.15. Choroid plexus of fourth ventricle

12.16. Deep cerebellar nuclei

12.17. Superior colliculus

For each numbered item, select the artery, or group of arteries, whose occlusion is most closely associated with the described syndrome. Each lettered heading may be selected once, more than once, or not at all.

Questions 12.18–12.22

(A) Paramedian branches of basilar artery
(B) Paramedian branches of basilar, posterior commuincating, and proximal posterior cerebral arteries
(C) Anterior spinal artery
(D) Short circumferential branches of basilar artery
(E) Branches of posterior communicating and posterior cerebral arteries

12.18. Middle alternating hemiplegia (Millard-Gubler syndrome)

12.19. Contralateral hemiballism

12.20. Superior alternating hemiplegia (Weber's syndrome)

12.21. Inferior alternating hemiplegia

12.22. Ipsilateral oculomotor palsy and contralateral cerebellar disturbances (Benedikt's syndrome)

For each numbered item, select the one heading most closely associated with it. Each lettered heading may be selected once, more than once, or not at all.

Questions 12.23–12.26

(A) Cervical spinal cord
(B) Thoracic spinal cord
(C) Lumbar spinal cord
(D) Conus medullaris
(E) Spinal epidural space

12.23. Internal vertebral venous plexus

12.24. Blood supply derived mainly from vertebral arteries

12.25. Arterial vasocorona

12.26. One unusually large anterior radicular artery

Questions 12.27–12.30

(A) Internal carotid artery
(B) Cerebral arterial circle
(C) Middle cerebral artery
(D) Anterior cerebral artery
(E) Basilar artery

12.27. Origin of anterior communicating artery

12.28. Origin of posterior communicating artery

12.29. Origin of posterior cerebral artery

12.30. Origin of anterior choroidal artery

Questions 12.31–12.34

(A) Superior sagittal sinus
(B) Rectus sinus
(C) Transverse sinus
(D) Cavernous sinus
(E) Basilar venous plexus

12.31. Contains the internal carotid artery

12.32. Receives the great vein of Galen

12.33. Arises from the confluens sinuum

12.34. Contains venous lacunae

Questions 12.35–12.38

(A) Cochlea
(B) Abducens nerve
(C) Trigeminal nerve
(D) Oculomotor nerve
(E) Optic nerve

12.35. Lies closest to internal carotid artery in the cavernous sinus

12.36. Supplied by a direct branch of the internal carotid artery

12.37. Passes between the superior cerebellar and posterior cerebral arteries

12.38. Supplied by a direct branch of the basilar artery

Questions 12.39–12.42

(A) Anterior perforated space
(B) Posterior perforated space
(C) Choroid plexus of third ventricle
(D) Nodulus and uvula of cerebellum
(E) Superior cerebellar peduncle

12.39. Medial posterior choroidal artery

12.40. Superior cerebellar artery

12.41. Lateral striate arteries

12.42. Branches of posterior communicating and posterior cerebral arteries

For each numbered item, indicate whether it is associated with

A only (A)
B only (B)
Both A and B (C)
Neither A or B (D)

Questions 12.43–12.46

(A) Anterior cerebral artery
(B) Middle cerebral artery
(C) Both
(D) Neither

12.43. Supplies primary motor and sensory cortex

12.44. Supplies the caudate nucleus and putamen

12.45. Supplies the visual cortex

12.46. Supplies the auditory cortex

Questions 12.47–12.50

(A) Anterior limb internal capsule
(B) Posterior limb internal capsule
(C) Both
(D) Neither

12.47. Lateral striate arteries

12.48. Medial striate artery

12.49. Anterior choroidal artery

12.50. Thalamogeniculate arteries

Questions 12.51–12.54

(A) Internal carotid artery
(B) Vertebral-basilar system
(C) Both
(D) Neither

12.51. Deep branches penetrate and supply the thalamus

12.52. Cervical portion gives rise to major arterial branches

12.53. Small direct branches supply trigeminal ganglion, tympanic cavity, and cavernous sinus

12.54. Supplies cochlea and vestibular apparatus

Questions 12.55–12.58

(A) Superficial cerebral veins
(B) Deep cerebral veins
(C) Both
(D) Neither

12.55. Run together with cerebral arteries

12.56. Drain directly or indirectly into the dural venous sinuses

12.57. Devoid of valves

12.58. Emissary veins

Questions 12.59–12.62

(A) Dural venous sinuses
(B) Superficial cerebral veins
(C) Both
(D) Neither

12.59. Anastomotic surface channels

12.60. Lined with endothelium

12.61. Emissary veins

12.62. Connections with deep cerebral veins

For each of the incomplete statements below, *one* or *more* of the completions given is correct. Choose answer:

(A) Only **1, 2,** and **3** are correct
(B) Only **1** and **3** are correct
(C) Only **2** and **4** are correct
(D) Only **4** is correct
(E) **All** are correct

12.63. The pontine tegmentum is supplied by:
(1) long circumferential branches of the basilar artery
(2) the anterior inferior cerebellar artery
(3) the superior cerebellar artery
(4) short circumferential branches of the basilar artery

12.64. Branches of the internal carotid artery include the:
(1) ophthalmic artery
(2) posterior communicating artery
(3) anterior choroidal artery
(4) anterior communicating artery

12.65. Arteries supplying the internal capsule include the:
(1) recurrent artery of Heubner
(2) middle cerebral artery
(3) anterior choroidal artery
(4) direct branches of the internal carotid artery

12.66. Bilateral occlusion of the anterior cerebral artery may produce:
(1) paresis in both lower extremities
(2) urinary incontinence
(3) sensory disturbances in lower limbs
(4) motor aphasia

12.67. The anterior choroidal artery:
(1) arises from the anterior cerebral artery
(2) supplies the retrolenticular part of the internal capsule
(3) supplies the medial thalamus
(4) supplies parts of both segments of the globus pallidus

12.68. The Sylvian triangle as seen in a lateral cerebral angiogram:
(1) contains branches of the middle cerebral artery
(2) contains the lenticulostriate arteries
(3) lies in the insula
(4) includes branches of the recurrent artery of Heubner

12.69. Occlusion of blood vessels supplying the midbrain tegmentum might produce:
(1) diplopia
(2) a small, unreactive pupil
(3) tremor and dysmetria
(4) lateral gaze paralysis

12.70. Branches of the posterior cerebral artery supply:
(1) parts of the inferior temporal gyrus
(2) the occipitotemporal and lingual gyri
(3) the cuneus
(4) the splenium of the corpus callosum

12.71. Spinal cord segments potentially most vulnerable to vascular lesions following interference with, or alterations of, segmental blood supply are:

(1) T4
(2) C8
(3) L1
(4) S3

12.72 Sudden occlusion of one posterior cerebral artery may produce:

(1) bilateral impairment of hearing
(2) loss of the pupillary light reflex
(3) heteronymous visual field defects
(4) contralateral homonymous hemianopsia

12.73. Complete or partial occlusion of the basilar artery may produce:

(1) diplopia
(2) vertigo and nystagmus
(3) dysarthria
(4) varying degrees of paresis on one or both sides

12.74. The internal cerebral vein receives blood from the:

(1) thalamostriate vein
(2) choroidal vein
(3) septal vein
(4) lateral ventricular vein

12.75. Veins draining bilaterally into the great vein of Galen include the:

(1) basal vein (Rosenthal)
(2) internal cerebral vein
(3) occipital vein
(4) posterior callosal vein

12.76. Cortical branches of the anterior cerebral artery supply the:

(1) orbital part of the frontal lobe
(2) paracentral gyrus
(3) cingulate gyrus
(4) cuneus

Answers and Explanations*

12.1. B An inferior alternating hemiplegia. See pp. 121 and 407

12.2. B See p. 18

12.3. D See p. 402

12.4. C See p. 404

12.5. C Branches of the middle cerebral artery frequently extend over the medial margin of the hemisphere and provide collateral circulation for the macular region of the striate cortex. See pp. 363 and 403

12.6. D See p. 399 and Fig. 14-5

12.7. E See p. 403 and Fig. 14-5

12.8. D See p. 404 and Fig. 14-8

12.9. A See p. 404 and Fig. 14-8

12.10. C See p. 407 and Fig. 14-14*B*

12.11. D See p. 403 and Fig. 14-5

12.12. E See p. 407 and Fig. 14-14*B*

12.13. A See p. 409 and Fig. 14-14*A*

12.14. B See p. 407 and Fig. 14-14*C*

12.15. C Medial branches of the posterior inferior cerebellar artery supply the choroid plexus of the fourth ventricle. See p. 411

12.16. D See p. 412. The anterior inferior cerebellar artery also supplies parts of the dentate nucleus

12.17. D See p. 410

12.18. A See pp. 155 and 409 as well as Fig. 14-14*A*

12.19. E Hemiballism usually results from a vascular lesion destroying parts of the subthalamic nucleus. The blood supply of this nucleus is derived from penetrating branches of the posterior communicating and posterior cerebral arteries

12.20. B Weber's syndrome involves the fibers of the oculomotor nerve and parts of the crus cerebri

12.21. C See pp. 121 and 407

12.22. B Benedikt's syndrome involves fibers of the oculomotor nerve, portions of the red nucleus, and surrounding fibers of the superior cerebellar peduncle above their decussation. See pp. 187–188

12.23. E See pp. 2 and 395; Fig. 41-3

12.24. A See p. 394

12.25. D See p. 394

12.26. C The artery of Adamkiewicz is a large anterior radicular artery found in the lumbar region

12.27. D See p. 398 and Fig. 14-4

12.28. A See p. 397 and Fig. 14-8

12.29. E See p. 402 and Figs. 14-4 and 14-8

12.30. A See p. 404 and Fig. 14-8

12.31. D The cavernous sinus contains the intracavernous segment of the internal carotid artery

12.32. B See p. 415 and Fig. 14-16

12.33. C See p. 412 and Fig. 1-3

12.34. A See p. 412 and Fig. 1-1

12.35. B The abducens nerve lies adjacent to the internal carotid artery in the cavernous sinus; see pp. 153 and 412

12.36. E The ophthalmic artery is a direct branch of cerebral segment of the internal carotid artery; see Fig. 14-4

12.37. D Both the trochlear and oculomotor nerves pass between the superior cerebellar and posterior cerebral arteries. An aneurysm of one of these arteries can produce pressure on the oculomotor nerve; see Fig. 14-4

12.38. A The labyrinthine artery

12.39. C The medial posterior choroidal artery is a branch of the posterior cerebral artery that supplies the choroid plexus of the third ventricle; see p. 404

* All page numbers and illustration citations refer to Carpenter: CORE TEXT OF NEUROANATOMY, 3rd edition; © 1985, Williams & Wilkins.

12.40. E The superior cerebellar artery supplies the superior cerebellar peduncle; see Fig. 14-14*A*

12.41. A See p. 404 and Figs. 12-2 and 14-8

12.42. B The posterior perforated space lies in the interpeduncular fossa; see p. 404

12.43. C See pp. 398–402 and Figs. 14-5 and 14-6

12.44. C See Fig. 14-9

12.45. D The possible except may be collaterals from the middle cerebral artery to the macular region

12.46. B See p. 402

12.47. C See p. 405

12.48. A See p. 405

12.49. B The anterior choroidal artery supplies the ventral and posterior part of the posterior limb of the internal capsule and the entire retrolenticular part; see Fig. 14-10

12.50. D The thalamogeniculate arteries supply the pulvinar and lateral thalamic nuclei, including the geniculate bodies; see p. 405

12.51. C The thalamus is supplied by the thalamoperforating and thalamogeniculate arteries derived from the posterior cerebral and from inferior thalamic arteries given off from the posterior communicating artery, a branch of the internal carotid artery

12.52. D Only small muscular branches are given off from the vertebral artery in its cervical course

12.53. A These small branches arise from the intracavernous part of the internal carotid artery

12.54. B The labyrinthine artery is a direct branch of the basilar artery; see p. 397 and Fig. 14-4

12.55. D Neither the superficial or deep cerebral veins course with cerebral arteries

12.56. C Both superficial and deep cerebral veins ultimately drain into the dural venous sinuses

12.57. D Neither have valves

12.58. D Neither have connections with extracranial veins via emissary veins

12.59. B Superficial veins lie in the pia mater and have numerous anastomotic channels on the surface; see p. 413

12.60. C Both are lined with endothelium

12.61. A The dural sinuses have connections with superficial veins of the scalp and head via emissary veins

12.62. C Both have connections with the deep cerebral veins; see p. 413

12.63. A See p. 409 and Fig. 14-14*A*

12.64. A See p. 395 and Figs. 14-4 and 14-8

12.65. E Se Fig. 14-10

12.66. A See p. 400

12.67. C See p. 404

12.68. B See pp. 400–401 and Fig. 14-7

12.69. B See p. 410

12.70. E See pp. 402–403

12.71. B See p. 394 and Fig. 14-1

12.72. D The calcarine arteries supply the visual cortex; see p. 403

12.73. E See p. 410

12.74. E See p. 414 and Fig. 14-19

12.75. A All are paired, except for the posterior callosal vein; which also drains into the great cerebral vein see p. 415

12.76. A The cortical branches of the anterior cerebral artery supply all listed structures except the cuneus, which is supplied by the branches of the posterior cerebral artery